*I'll Be OK, It's Just a Hole in My Head*

*A Memoir on Heartbreak and Head Trauma*

By Mimi Hayes

*I'll Be OK, It's Just a Hole in My Head*
*A Memoir on Heartbreak and Head Trauma*
Copyright © 2018

Animal Media Group books may be ordered through booksellers, or by contacting:

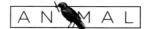

Animal Media Group
100 1ˢᵗ Ave suite 1100
Pittsburgh, PA 15222
animalmediagroup.com
(412) 566-5656

ISBN: 978-1-947895-04-1 (pbk)
ISBN: 978-1-947895-05-8 (ebk)

Susan Holmes!

OT for the win! Thank you for everything you do for our community! You rock! ♡

♡ Miss Hayes

**Praise for *I'll Be OK, It's Just a Hole in My Head***

"Mimi has the unique ability to exist outside of herself and write about what she went through as though she were floating above it all, watching with mixed horror and fascination. But her humor and wit are always there to hold the reader's hand, reminding you that everything will (maybe?) be okay."

— Adam Clayton-Holland, *Those Who Can't, Conan*

"Mimi takes us on her own voyage into the human brain, in a uniquely touching and humorous way. Highly recommended for anyone interested in the most vital of all organs!"

— Lotje Sodderland, *My Beautiful Broken Brain*

"Mimi takes the reader on a journey through her tragedy authentically and vulnerably, which is no small feat. Her voice is fresh, clever, and downright motivational. This book should be required reading for anyone experiencing trauma or the unexpected obstacles of life."

— Gregg Clunis, *Tiny Leaps, Big Changes*

"Mimi might have a hole in her head, but this book will put a hole in your heart. But don't worry! I mean that in a good way. And besides, Mimi will then fill that hole with laughs. For a mix of delightful humor and poignant thoughts on the obstacles that we encounter in life, please read this book."

— Nate Dern, *Not Quite a Genius*

For my Momsie and Popsicle.
The first people to ever love me. And my #1 fans.


Also for my ex-boyfriend. I bet this is awkward.


More importantly, for Bernard and Peggy.
I miss you every single day.

# Table of Contents:

# Prologue

*Friday, September 5, 2014, 11:20 p.m.*

INT. SAINT JOSEPH HOSPITAL EMERGENCY ROOM

MIMI lies on the examination table. She emerged from the "metal donut" several minutes ago and now is resting in the room with MOM. She is tired and trying to sleep. MOM sits close to her and strokes her hair. The lights are dimmed. NURSE comes back into the room with her tiny brown clipboard and turns to MOM.

NURSE:

We found something.

MOM sits up, alarmed. The plastic curtains sway backward as if taking impact from the information. MIMI remains motionless. NURSE addresses MOM.

NURSE:

A part of your daughter's brain is bleeding—

MOM looks horrified. Her mouth hangs ajar. MIMI does not move or blink. NURSE moves to the door quickly.

NURSE:

I'm going to make a phone call. Please wait here.

NURSE leaves the room for an undisclosed location. MOM looks to MIMI. MIMI'S eyes are wide open and focused on the ceiling tiles. Her mouth moves slightly as if she is counting them. MIMI shivers, her body convulsing, like she's trying to find warmth. MOM grabs a blanket from behind her and covers MIMI. MIMI'S skin has turned translucent.

MOM:

Shh. You're okay. You're okay.

MIMI continues to shiver. MOM grabs another blanket and puts it atop MIMI. MOM strokes MIMI'S hair.

MOM:

You're okay—

"—CUT!" Steven Spielberg screams. He throws his weathered director's hat on the ground and calls for the makeup people to come retouch my face, because beads of sweat are running into my eyes and ruining my eyeliner. As they dab orange goo onto my forehead, Spielberg approaches.

"What are you, cold or something?" He props one hand on his hip in agitation.

"W-what?" I say.

"The shivering. It looks weird on camera. I need to see the pain *in your eyes.* Candace, can we get her a blanket or something? This is ridiculous…

"Mom, you're doing great. I like the 'you're okay' line. Very inventive. Nurse, nice exit. Get out of there as soon as you can, almost with no explanation at all—in fact, yes, let's try that this time. Just come in, say the brain is bleeding, then run out the door. Skip that whole making a phone call line."

Spielberg trudges back to his director's chair. He dramatically snatches his hat from the ground and places it back upon his simmering head. "RESET."

A swift set crew emerges from the curtains to move me slightly back on the examination table. They tuck blankets around me, jabbing me in the side as they haphazardly try to cure me of my shivers. Their efforts prove unsuccessful. I am still fucking freezing. The nurse takes two steps back out of frame.

"ROLLING…"

"ACTION!"

…There I go again. Trying to turn my life into a Hollywood blockbuster. It's a very bad habit I've developed, you guys.

This didn't happen. Not even a little bit. There was no cutting or resetting. Spielberg wasn't in that emergency room to give actor's notes or to yell at me for shivering in a 95-degree room. I didn't have unlimited access to blankets or stage makeup. Because this wasn't a movie scene: this was my life. And try as I might to fantasize my way out of it, *I was not okay.*

## Noodly Rowboats

I'm not a scientist. I'm not a psychologist, a neurologist, or a brain surgeon. But I know that my brain is all kinds of messed up. It's gooey in there. I did the math. And it turns out I'm not very good at math either. I've done word problems that ask me to calculate who's on first and how many groceries they have in their basket after a train departs at ten. I bump into every door frame that presents itself to me, and every morning at six o'clock I take my medication and then forget if I took it.

If I tell you a story, it's likely you've heard it before, and if I tell you a story, it's likely you've heard it before. I make peach and mango protein smoothies because they remind me of when Rosie tried to help me get my leg muscles back. I once spent a whole five minutes on an electronic bull, throwing a medicine ball back and forth with my therapist. I should mention that this particular electronic bull moved in slow motion. And that I only got the ball to the face twelve times.

My mother likes to show off my scar. She takes pride in thrusting my head at friends or at strangers at the grocery store and throwing back my hair. "Look at this, see? All the way down, it goes all the way down. *That's where they went in*," she says maniacally.

Sometimes when I roll over in bed too fast, a tiny part of my stomach does backflips, and I have to exhale a bit to remember that I'm in my bed and not on a teacup ride. If I'm in a large crowd for too long, I will create an escape plan in my head for when I inevitably start hyperventilating and panicking. Coffee shops are fine for a few hours, until I get tired and the sound of an espresso machine resembles a blow horn. If I attend too many meetings, words will jumble together and make no sense. I can take a nap absolutely anywhere and nowhere if it's too loud.

I drive a car, drink alcohol, and don't get a handicapped parking space. I should clarify: I don't drive a car and drink alcohol *at the same time*. I'm just saying these are two separate things I am able to do as a functioning human. I can even perform exciting tasks like brush my own teeth, tie my shoes, and correctly use a toaster oven. Also, I'm a little bitter about the handicapped parking situation. I guess having been in a wheelchair for eight days two years ago doesn't actually qualify me for that front spot at Chipotle. Who knew?

I wasn't always the lopsided mess I appear to be today. Before the CAT scans, MRIs, and hospital pudding, I was just like all of you fine people. Completely and totally normal. Except for a small delusion at bedtime that I was actually Snow White waiting to be brought back to life and that there'd never be a shortage of cherry pies for my dwarfs to eat while I lay peacefully in my temporary coma.

I grew up in the land of '90s Disney plot holes. My parents called me their little princess, and everything was magical in the confines of my perfectly intact mind. I spent hours on trampolines and in trees, except I wasn't jumping or climbing, oh goodness, no. I was reclaiming land grants from the evil king of France or masquerading as an undercover Russian spy. Shit, I could've grown tentacles and slunk away into the ocean with a talking hand puppet named Clarence if I really wanted to. And you know, maybe I should. Because that sounds like an awful lot of fun.

I continued to live in a cocoon of imagination long past an acceptable age. My imagination wove itself into my relationships, my choices, and my neurons. The grown-ups might call this denial. I called it Mimi's Awesome Land of Make-Believe and Avoiding Adult Responsibilities.

It didn't occur to me then that my head was broken before it was broken—that I desperately needed a brain overhaul. Oh, I got one all right. Just not the one I expected. But before I can tell you what my gooey brain looks like now, we have to go back to the beginning. Or rather, the beginning of the end.

James was my guy.

At seventeen, I could hardly manage my thick, curly locks or rambunctious spirit, but I was ready for my guy to sweep me off my tiny feet, love me for all my quirks, and call me his girl. I didn't know then that I'd lose him down the road. As far as my young, curly head was concerned, we'd be together forever.

The sweltering summer sun blasted through the car window, and I shifted in my seat. We were en route to another family reunion, this one in my aunt's cabin in the mountains of Grand Lake, Colorado.

"Aren't you going to be hot?" my little brother, Brian, asked. He poked at my heavy black sweater, knitted hat, and tight bell-bottoms. My older sister, Erin, was too preoccupied with her headphones to concern herself with my outfit choice.

"We're going to the *mountains*," I said. "It's cold up there." He had a point. It was the middle of July, and underneath my black hat was a matted ring of sweaty hair. My frontal lobe was still developing along with my hat head.

When two hours later, we pulled into the drive of Aunt Karen's beautiful mountain home, I was kicking Brian and Erin in the shins—likely a symptom of heatstroke. *Get me out of this car, oh my god, I'm done with you people.* The air was crisp and hot, the smell of barbeque lingering.

Mom hugged her sisters and waved at us kids. "Go make yourselves useful. And get the dog out of the car, for goodness' sake." We'd left Tucker in the back panting.

"Sorry, buddy," I said, petting his shaggy head.

As we unloaded the coolers, chairs, and canine, a boy who looked vaguely familiar stepped out from the garage to help us. He stood six feet, a good foot taller than I was. I loved the height difference and immediately decided everyone would be jealous of our adorable and imaginary love affair. He was lanky, but in a cute, artistic way. I imagined him in an art studio throwing paint at the wall with his strong hands. His smile might light up a room; his laugh would fill it. His chocolate-brown eyes reminded me of, well, chocolate. I dreamed of rolling his hair into little ringlets with my fingers. From the second I saw him, I knew he was my guy.

Within minutes, I'd constructed an intricate future with this stranger. I'd planted the seed of a fantasy love affair. Laughing together in a rowboat, long walks on the beach by the ocean—wait, what the hell was I thinking? I lived in a landlocked state. And a *rowboat*? This is what the brain can do. It can weave you and your petite rowboat into a complex, fantastical web. Like a big bowl of spaghetti noodles; a never-ending mess of noodly rowboat make-believe.

He grabbed a chair from me, and our eyes met for the first time.

I felt as if I'd known those large, chocolate chip eyes all my life. It turns out I did know him. Our families had been acquainted since my birth. This was the little boy I had sat next to on a wagon at the zoo and on a picnic blanket circa 1996. We hadn't seen each other since age nine or ten.

The car door slammed shut, sending me out of my spaghetti noodle trance.

I smiled as he headed up the stairs to the patio. "I'm Mimi," I said to his back.

"James, nice to meet you," he called. Even from the back of his disheveled head, I could feel his smile.

By the end of the day, I was in deep. I followed him around the party all evening, desperately imagining a reality in which James could fall in love with me too. When we exchanged numbers, I held my phone as though it were the most sacred thing my hands would touch. I'd have left a shoe for him to find on the back porch like Cinderella, but that might have been weird.

Two weeks after the cabin, we met up for our first real date. It was at Water World, an amusement park and Colorado treasure.

"So…where do we go from here?" I asked coyly as we rounded the corner between the water slides and the tidal wave pool. *Oh please, oh please, oh please ask me to be your girlfriend.* I clenched my fists into tiny balls, awaiting his answer; did my prince think that my sweaty flip-flop was worth saving?

"I thought we could hit up the Dinosaur ride and then go back around to the Lazy River."

"I meant…with you and me," I said, feeling like Cinderella's ugly twin.

"Oh! Well, you're…"

I held my breath, bracing for impact.

"…my girlfriend now," he said with a smile. My hands relaxed, and he planted a kiss on my nervous lips. Love was as simple and carefree as the Lazy River.

We began dating our senior year of high school, and the world seemed like it was ours for the taking. James was as artistic and charming as my rowboat fantasy hoped he'd be. He was a budding photographer and enjoyed snapping pictures with his old-timey cameras wherever we went. He was crafty. He made me homemade gifts like a Lego radio and flowers created from recycled soda pop cans.

"Can you believe how cute this guy is?" I'd say to my friends, passing around my Pepsi, Sprite, and Orange Crush bouquet.

James was spontaneous, like any good Disney prince. His top surprises included stapling roses to the walls of my classrooms, along with encrypted notes about where to find my next clue (a.k.a. the next class in my schedule), and planning weekend getaways to tiny mountain towns during the spring and summer. He'd throw his wrinkly hands over my eyes and lead me forward.

"Where are we going?" I'd ask.

"You'll see."

He showed me his beat-up truck. Not a chariot, but it would do nicely. Once he got his driver's license, we roamed the long dirt roads by his house and watched the sun go down among the weeds and wildflowers. We'd listen to country music, and he'd coo along to the beat as he held my hand. I lived for these drives. Saying goodbye could take an hour some nights, us lingering in his truck as the stars came out, and kissing and then coming back for more. We almost always broke our curfews. Had my fantasy been historically accurate, I would have turned into a pumpkin.

Everything seemed so easy and natural. My fairy tale was real. I said, "I love you" on Halloween, a mere two months into dating James. I could tell him anything: my fear of the unknown, and my obsession with sharks and knickknacks. Nothing in the world could stop us from having our own little happily ever after. It didn't matter that we were landlocked. We'd row ourselves into the sunset on our very own boat made of penne.

## Heartbreak at 14,000 Feet

After high school I planned to play college ice hockey. Throughout my childhood my mother had tried to gently guide me toward a path better suited to my body type—you know, miniature—but it was no use. My father had played at the University of Denver, and his princess had a pair of ice skates and wanted to play in the big leagues too.

There were no Division I, II, or III women's teams in Colorado. I'd known this for a while; I'd been researching women's college teams since my sophomore year of high school. I didn't want to leave James, but I worried that I would be giving up on my dream of college sports if I stayed. I didn't want to be one of those girls who stayed for a guy. Think of all the dope places the Little Mermaid could have run off to once she got those new legs, instead of hanging around that Prince Eric all the time. Besides, I thought our relationship was stronger than that.

When I started looking at colleges in the Midwest, James was supportive, but he hugged me tighter every time I talked about leaving. My insides battled like a hockey fight in the pit of my stomach. On one side was my lifelong dream. And on the other, my growing love for James. Ultimately hockey won me over.

I set my sights on a small liberal arts college in Minnesota, the College of Saint Benedict and Saint John's University. Then I went out for a visit and fell in love with the tiny college town and friendly people. When I met with the coach, he said I'd have a place on the team if I came out in the fall.

"This is the one," I told James. I'd called him from the Mall of America as my mother and I wandered the food court.

"That's great, baby. You should do it." But underneath his happy tone, I could hear the pain.

Meanwhile, James had started thinking about his future too. He was excited about enrolling in photography classes at the community college. He didn't want to take out loans, so he decided to pay for school as he went.

"You can go wherever you want!" I said one day. "Aren't there some pretty cool photography programs around?"

"Easy for you to say."

I squirmed in my seat.

"My mom can't cosign a loan for me." A tiny surge of resentment hit me across the airwaves for the very first time since we started dating. My parents had been saving for my college years since before I was born, twenty-five bucks a month even when they didn't have it. I'd still be paying off student loans my whole life, but their support would ease the burden once I graduated and began making loan payments. His dad had split when he was a kid, leaving his mom to care for him and his younger sister. James had grown up in a trailer park. He hadn't had the same opportunities I'd had as a child. I'd never considered myself spoiled or rich, but in his eyes I might as well have had a silver spoon hanging from my mouth.

When we graduated high school, we agreed to date long distance and make it work a thousand miles apart. I didn't know it then, but I was testing our relationship. If he stuck with me throughout my hockey dreams, then we'd get married for sure. Minnesota would be my litmus test. I was donning fancy scientist gloves and preparing to test my hypothesis: *we are made for each other.*

How was it possible that two teenagers thought they could beat the geographical gods and breeze through four years of long-distance dating unscathed? Ah, the misapprehensions and sheer overconfidence of first love. You know it well. We didn't. Neither of us could emotionally handle breaking up and didn't want to. We decided to stay together and let the rest magically take care of itself.

"I love you so much," I cried after we'd packed my last boxes into the Tahoe. I considered leaving a shoe behind just to see if he'd follow me.

"You have to do this, I know," he said.

He picked me up and carried my sobbing self to the car. Suddenly I wasn't ready. Why was I leaving this boy I loved so much for some stupid sport? Had I gone completely delusional?

We pulled away from the house, and I watched him standing on the porch until he disappeared from view. I cried all the way through Wyoming.

Making it work didn't work as well as we'd thought it would. As school started up and hockey season began, we had less time to talk on the phone or Skype. It became easier to bicker at each other in frustration. I tried to convince my roommate, Sami, that this was the man I was going to marry someday. I'd even picked the cake, I told her. It would be made of donuts, because I saw it on Pinterest once. The long-distance squabbling was just a phase that we'd grow out of, like our frozen yogurt addiction last summer.

"You guys fight on the phone constantly," she said. "I could hear you crying in the hallway last night."

That was a new habit. There was nowhere else I could go. I didn't want to be outside in the lobby for everyone to see, and I didn't want to bug Sami by sobbing on our bunk beds. Our dorm had a strange enclosure with a glass door in the center of the hall, just tight enough to squeeze into. If I fell asleep there sniffling into my phone, I would look like Snow White; my hallmates could serve as my dwarfs. Somehow I was much more concerned with not looking like a lunatic in Dorm Corona D Wing than I was with ending every phone call to my boyfriend in tears.

During these late-night calls, I'd guilt James about not taking a more rigorous class schedule. It upset me that I was balancing a full course load, three hours of hockey practice a day, and a long-distance boyfriend, while he was working at a factory and deciding not to go to the big photography school in California. He'd guilt me about moving away in the first place.

"I can't Skype this weekend—we'll be in Wisconsin for a tournament," I told him over the phone one evening while packing my bags for another hockey trip.

"Fine, whatever. I see how it is." His words hit me like a bitter wind.

"It's not that I don't want to!" I said. "I have practice for three hours, and I have to write this history paper before our games…" I felt like I was walking on a thin sheet of Minnesotan ice.

The guilting continued. If a good thing was happening in one of our lives, it was shit for the other. If I did well on a history final, he'd become bitter about his job at the electroplating factory. When he got into an art show, I'd be upset about not getting ice time.

For years I'd held on to the hope that I could be good enough to play in the Olympics someday. I wanted to be Sara DeCosta-Hayes, who isn't related to me but was the star goalie for the 1998 gold medal and the 2002 silver. But maybe I wasn't destined to play college sports or in the Olympics. Maybe I'd made a huge mistake. Princesses didn't leave their princes like that, at least not in this patriarchal fairy tale of mine. I needed James to support me in what had been the most important part of my life for the past decade. But he couldn't, at least not in the way I needed him to. I considered buying a flight home immediately.

Sami and a few of my friends from the hall planned an intervention, but it was too late; I was leaving Minnesota and going back to Colorado. I told a few friends in secret. I went on a long run to clear my mind the day I made my decision.

I put my Pandora radio on shuffle and plugged in my earphones on the Quad. I remember feeling like every song was speaking to me. Amos Lee sang of the one he couldn't stay away from, and his cooing soothed my ripping heart. James was still my guy. It was one of those moments that puts your whole life into perspective—or so I thought at the time. Perspective can be deceiving, especially when your brain stops working and you end up with double vision. But we'll get to that later.

After a hard year apart, serious soul searching, and reading too much into romantic lyrics, I quit hockey and transferred home to Colorado. If hockey wasn't going to work out, I had better get back to my landlocked fairy tale. I could live with not being the star athlete I'd hoped to be if it meant I kept my guy.

And we were ready to mend what had felt broken for ten months. I was burned out from being a college athlete. He was just happy we were in the same time zone. The bickering subsided, and we spent almost every day together again. I enrolled at the University of Colorado at Boulder, and he took classes sporadically at local community colleges. I took up college improv; he built a longboard. We were back to spontaneous car rides, now to new destinations like Rocky Mountain National Park and Moab, Utah. We were young and stupid and back in love. On our third anniversary, he gave me a promise ring.

Soon my donut cake would be a reality.

I switched my focus from sports to teaching and threw myself into my studies. I was moving in an intentional direction—I had found my new purpose. I'd walk away with a teaching license in a few years. With James, it wasn't so easy to tell. He was accepted to a prestigious photography institute—twice—and turned it down—twice. He enrolled in college but would only take one class per semester. I thought his talent and potential were being wasted, and I had no qualms telling him so. He grew more resentful about my opinion on his education. We belittled each other 24/7/365.

James made it clear that I was not as ready for my new career as I thought I was. "You don't know anything about history," he said one evening as I was studying my notes. "You can't even remember the names of Civil War heroes or World War II fighter planes. How could you possibly be a history teacher?"

I buried my face in my worn copy of *World War II in Asia and the Pacific* and sobbed. I felt as if he didn't believe in a fundamental part of me. Not only did he find Teaching Me hilariously inept, but also College Feminist Me, Hockey-Playing Me, and sometimes Spoiled Princess Me. He'd reluctantly come to see Improv Me in *The Vagina Monologues* but didn't sit with my mother and rejected my invitation to take him to the afterparty to meet all my cool feminist friends.

He was always working, but I could never understand what he was working toward. We weren't just on different pages; we were wandering in different libraries. The bright-eyed boy I'd known back in high school was gone. He started working eighteen-hour shifts back to back as a ramp agent at the airport. It was my senior year then, and I was still living in Boulder finishing up school. We hardly saw each other, and when we did, he was tired or angry. Even the few times we traveled together with his flight benefits—Paris, Rome, and San Francisco—he wasn't happy, treating me more like a wife he wanted to divorce than a girlfriend he wanted to marry.

James began picking up shifts on Christmas and holidays to avoid being around my family. He flew to Australia on a whim on Valentine's Day—without me. I spent the day sobbing with a friend on the couch and then later in public at a nice Italian restaurant. Then again on the couch.

He even made a big fuss about attending my college graduation. "I don't see why I have to be there," he said. "I told my friend I would go to Japan with him that weekend."

"It's my *graduation*. Why are you being so weird about this?" I set my coffee cup down on my cracked kitchen counter. He'd helped me move into this old college house for my senior year, along with every small apartment and cramped home I'd lived in the past few years. My gaze wandered to the walls, where the wallpaper had been painted over several times. The peeling white walls were so grungy compared with the perfectly built little castles in my brain. Those castles were now crumbling.

I stared down into my black coffee. My rage was brewing and would surely boil over into my mug, my anger turned into dark-roasted, hazelnut-flavored fury. It would go great with my burned bagel and expired cream cheese.

In an effort to fix our rotting wallpaper relationship, I found a couple's survey online for us to complete. Questions like "I feel respected when we do _____ together" focused on the positive while helping the couple analyze issues and look for solutions. If we couldn't do this, my fairy tale was a lie. If we couldn't talk about our relationship, maybe there wasn't a relationship at all. After nearly five years of carefully constructed fantasies and ideas collected on a Pinterest wedding board, I didn't very much like the idea of no donut cake wedding, but I was unable to envision it now as my near future.

I filled out my questionnaire in January of my senior year and hinted for James to do his part for months. My feebleness became routine. I lost the ability to communicate. And this was *before* my brain injury rendered me speech impaired.

"Did you get around to that survey?" I'd say like a tiny mouse.

"I'll do it later."

"No rush!" And I'd smile to hide my disappointment.

I mailed a copy of the questionnaire to him in March, willing myself to believe that he would open it and recognize how important it was to me. In my mind, he would complete it immediately. I couldn't come right out and tell him that this survey meant the very life and death of our relationship. I kept that part to myself.

For the next few months I prepared for graduation. I set up meetings with schools for my student teaching semester and told myself that this stressful time with James would soon pass. I had a promise ring. My fantasy could still exist. If he completed the survey, we could have a real come-to-Jesus moment and emerge from our funk. I'd be lying if I said I wasn't hoping for a scene out of a '90s chick flick. Probably *Jerry Maguire*.

One afternoon in April he said he had to see me. That sounded either utterly sweet or dangerously bad. Maybe I was getting my *Jerry* scene after all. Or maybe I was getting that scene from *My Girl* with the fucking bees. I went home and changed into a casually cute outfit and stuffed some Kleenex in my purse just in case.

Because even though a breakup scene wasn't in my dream world's screenplay, I could feel it in my bones. He'd grown distant over the past few months. He'd hide his phone from me, acting suspiciously, then do sweet things out of the blue.

"Have you seen my boyfriend?" I'd asked our friend Moe one night as we rounded another corner together on our group bike ride. I was pretty used to James not biking next to me during these outings, but it seemed unusual that the pack had remained together on the bike ride, and James and a girl named Molly were missing most of the night.

Moe's lips tightened. It was clear to both of us what was going on, or at least it should have been. But I wouldn't have seen it coming—not even if James had made a gigantic intervention sign that read "Seriously, not going to marry you!" I had my head so deep in imagination land that I questioned what was real and what was make-believe.

In the dim light of the coffee shop that April afternoon, James said, "We're just different people now. We're growing apart, and I—"

"I'm not a different person now. I'm the same person." The café was packed, and he'd been almost an hour late. Was this seriously happening right now? In a public place, no less?

"It sounds a lot like you're breaking up with me." My coffee tasted like poison in my mouth.

"I'm not!"

"Okay?" I stifled my sobs inside my cup and checked to see if anyone else in the café had seen what almost happened.

These stupid conversations continued for a month until he finally ripped off the Band-Aid in May. In hindsight, it must have been the hardest thing he'd ever had to do. It was one of the only times I'd seen him cry.

This was Monday, May 19, 2014, two days after my college graduation. After three hours of studying plant-based diets during the rationing years of World War II for my teacher licensure exam and eight hours of playing the name game with all the new lifeguards at the summer camp where I worked, I was exhausted. I called James in desperate need of some cuddles and wine. I wish I didn't remember this night with such vivid detail. Darn you, future hemorrhage! Why couldn't you have happened in my *temporal* lobe?

We met in the parking lot of a random restaurant on the outskirts of Denver near midnight. I looked up at James in relief, glad to be together after such a long day. He was smiling with pity, almost as if at an injured deer that he'd just hit with his car. I couldn't forget it if I tried.

"You're going to hate me," he said.

My silly rowboat-obsessed heart sank. *Abandon ship, we're going down!* I knew right away I was going to need more than the three Kleenex in my purse. He insisted we go inside the restaurant and sit down. I refused and headed directly back to my car. If this was really happening, then I sure as hell wasn't going to sob in front of Kimberly, "the newest waitstaff to the Chili's family." Her name could have been Holly or Candace, I didn't give a shit; she was not going to see me cry.

We sat in my car for two and a half hours as he broke my heart into tiny pieces. He "needed to find himself." He'd "lost his way." I didn't understand. He was sitting right beside me. How the hell could he be lost? I knew where he was. And I knew who he was—he was my guy.

"Maybe I'll just miss you too much and come back," he said.

"Give this back to me when you mean it," I said, handing him the promise ring. Then I gave him one last snot-covered kiss. I hope he tasted every single one of those boogers.

I went through the rest of my week in denial. Maybe I wasn't a Disney princess; maybe I was Rocky Balboa. I'd just taken a punch to the kisser. Now I'd come back swinging. I showed up at his doorstep at four o'clock in the morning several days later and threw rocks at his window. I could see him through the window, ignoring my calls.

He finally came outside. His jaw was clenched tight along with his hands.

Questions fogged my brain. *Are you seeing someone else? Is she in your bed right now? Shit, is it that nineteen-year-old Molly chick? Are you just going to walk out after nearly five years, with no explanation other than some "I have to go find myself" bullshit?*

He answered none of these questions and told me to leave.

~

I sat on my parents' couch, sobbing. It was June 15, a Sunday. I stared down at the Instagram photograph on my phone in despair and contemplated the likelihood that my phone would shatter if I hurled it at the wall. The chances were good, but I considered it all the same. I buried my face in my mother's plush red pillow and screamed. The photo was a selfie my very recent ex-boyfriend had taken with his very new girlfriend atop Quandary Peak, a Colorado fourteener.

Just nine months earlier I had taken a similar selfie atop the same mountain with James on our four-year anniversary. The first and only fourteener I had ever climbed, and I was proud of it too. Climbing up jagged rock faces for hours on end was not something I'd ever seen myself doing, but when I got to the top, I felt like a champion. The real Rocky. We'd packed sandwiches and chocolate bars and ate them at the top of the world, a magnificent landscape stretching before us.

To recap: he took her to *our* anniversary spot. And posted it on Instagram for the world to see. For me to see. I choked on my tears and screamed some more into Mom's pillow.

The breakup was done in such an epic and public manner that my mother knew about it even before I told her. Thanks to social media, he made sure to let his new gal pal post pictures of their romantic date nights on everyone's news feed just days after the breakup. Prince Charming, you guys. I was a mess.

I gawked at every Facebook update and Instagram picture and hated them both. It was toxic. Worst of all, I noticed a tiny piece of me in everything they did together, almost as if he was repeating our relationship with her. He took her to our restaurants. His chocolate-brown eyes were now fixed on her. He cuddled up next to her in one photo, wearing the Saint John's T-shirt I'd bought him. I felt deceived, embarrassed, and small. I couldn't accept that my best friend would so easily turn his back on me. All our inside jokes, the moments we shared, the things that only we knew about each other—and he had walked away from it all as if it never existed. As if *I* never existed.

Maybe James had been my guy. But I wasn't his girl.

## Berlitz

When I was young, I was fascinated by my grandfather's French Canadian heritage. My great-great-grandparents Octavia and Odilon Gagnon (fancy names, *non?*) hailed from Quebec and brought their family down to Lake Linden, Michigan. Omar Gagnon, my great-grandfather, was born there on August 9, 1873. Omar's son, Bernard Gagnon—my darling Papa—grew up in Campbell, Nebraska, where the family moved alongside many other French Canadians.

Our family get-togethers were always spent in the Gagnon basement. A tablecloth covering the large Ping-Pong table glistened with steaming platters of homemade food. There was the kids' table too, a pop-up table tacking on to the back of the TV room. But I never had to sit at the kids' table, because I always had my own seat next to Papa, right by the head of the table. I didn't even mind that I had to sit on five phonebooks just to make eye contact with my food. I was the favorite, and everyone knew it.

The Gagnons of Campbell, Nebraska, continued to speak French throughout my grandpa's life, which I thought was just awesome. I can still remember my grandmother telling me how terrified she was to meet my grandfather's family for the first time. She entered a crowded kitchen full of fast-talking French people and couldn't understand a damn word they were saying. By the time I knew him, my grandfather had lost most of the language, but I thought he'd come around to it again if I started speaking to him. In sixth grade, I signed up for French classes so that I could talk to Papa and reconnect with my French roots.

Fast-forward to a few months into my French learning. I wasn't very good, but I told Papa how excited I was to speak to him in his native tongue. *J'ai hâte de parler avec toi.* One day he gave me a gift. He went down to their dusty old grandparenty basement and pulled out a little Berlitz French travel book from the 1940s. It was adorable, with its tiny beret-wearing American dancing around the pages and its tips on how to find the bathroom or order at restaurants. *Où est la toilette? Bonjour, je m'appelle Mimi.* It was, and continues to be, my single most important possession.

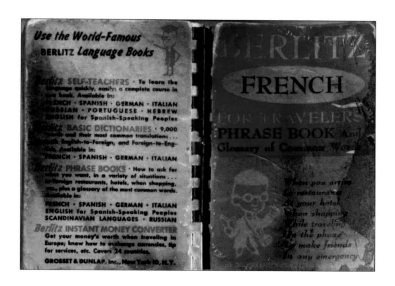

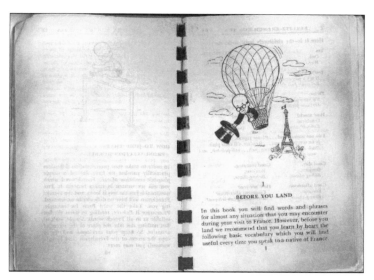

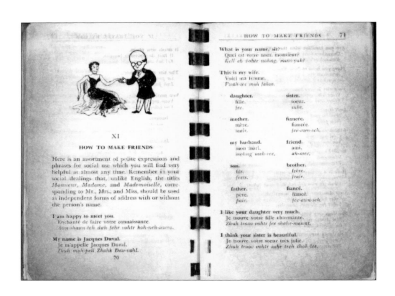

My grandfather, Bernard Omar Gagnon, gave me this gift in August 2004. He passed away shortly after.

When he passed away, the only thing I had left of him was the Berlitz French book. And in the first year of my relationship with James, I gave it away. I was so in love that I gave James my most sacred possession. *Here's this thing that means everything to me; let's be together forever.* Maybe I considered it a dowry, I don't know.

It was certainly a risk to entrust this family relic to a new love. You'd think my brain had already exploded. James moved almost every six months, so it's a small miracle that it made it through so many travels.

But then came the opportunity of a lifetime: a trip to the holy land, Paris, France! James was working at the airport, so we could travel cheap by flying standby. It would be the first of many trips across the pond for us, but for this inaugural adventure I wanted only one thing: to bring old Berlitz to France and reconnect with Papa. We unearthed the book from a box in storage and brought him along for the adventure.

The trip was short, a mere five days crammed full of trips to the Louvre, boat tours around the Eiffel Tower, and a train ride to the Palace of Versailles. We were both sick the entire time with a head cold we'd picked up on the flight over, so we were quite grumpy. James wouldn't smile in pictures and seemed peeved at my jolly-romping, almost like it was a chore that we were in France. But I still can't put into words the excitement I felt being there, giggly with my Berlitz.

When we got home from our illness-riddled Paris adventure, Berlitz stayed buried in his travel bag for months.

"Have you seen Berlitz?" I said one evening over spaghetti.

"What?" He was tired and snappy.

"The French book?"

"Look in my bag, I don't know."

I dug through his bag to find that a bottle of sunscreen had committed suicide beside my dear Berlitz and turned him bright blue, sticking his poor little French pages together. I was devastated that I'd left my most prized possession alone in a crummy bag instead of standing him proudly on a shelf. I couldn't believe I'd taken my eyes off Berlitz for a second.

It didn't occur to me then, but I'd sacrificed Berlitz. Over the course of the relationship, I'd given away more and more in hopes of a happily ever after with James. Berlitz wasn't just a book or a knickknack. Berlitz was my grandfather, my friend, a connection to my past and my history. I'd abandoned that part of myself.

James was unaffected by the incident. "It's fine," he said.

I foraged for a paper towel and patted down the pages.

~

After several weeks of post-breakup delusions, James and I reconnected. But now I'd decided to stop fooling myself. It was time for the exchange of shit.

The shit-collecting process can be difficult on both parties. And when you've been together nearly five years, there's a lot of shit. But at that moment, all I wanted back was the book, so that's all I asked for from James.

The day came for the exchange. I put his clothes, bike, and phone chargers on the porch and made a mad dash to get down the block so I wouldn't have to be there when he picked them up. He could leave my things at the door. Then his truck rounded the corner, and I swallowed my pride with a big gulp.

"Just put everything over there." I pointed to the corner of the porch and avoided his chocolate-brown eyes.

I loaded his rubbish into the back of his truck to speed up the process. He fumbled through the cab and unearthed everything I'd ever given him: bags of love letters, pictures of us, old gifts, sticky notes, all of it. He rummaged around more and accidentally knocked my homemade Christmas box onto the street. Small trinkets fell to the cement and scattered.

*Why don't you just run over it with your truck a few times, then take a gigantic shit all over it?* But I wanted to treat him with some of the dignity and respect that he hadn't shown me. I also wanted to punch his teeth out. He was cold, callous, even angry at me. Looking back, I realize this process must have been hard on him and his new lady. If I were waiting months for *my* new boyfriend to dump his longtime girlfriend, I'd probably be pretty uptight about having all that stuff around too.

I wanted closure aside from my pile of belongings. Closure to me was comforting words, not a bag of old clothes and love letters that I hadn't asked for. There was even a bright blue bouncy ball in a box. No idea where the fuck that had come from. I clutched it tightly like a stress ball.

"Are you okay?" I asked.

"I better bite my lip," he said.

"What is that supposed to mean?"

"I just better bite my lip." *Well, that's strange*, I thought, *aren't you the one with the other girlfriend on the side, the one walking out after five years?* He was speaking as if I was the one who had ripped his heart out and taken a glorious piss on it.

I later found out that my father had texted him after hearing about Molly.

> Dad: Listen, Shit Stain. I know exactly what you did. And if you so much as think about showing your face around our family, I will kill you where you stand.
>
> James (a.k.a. "Shit Stain"): I was just doing the right thing.
>
> Dad: Having another relationship on the side is not "the right thing" and you damn well know it. Stay away. Also go fuck yourself.

When you mess with Daddy's little girl, you get a sniper rifle to the head, not a warm hug. You are messing with the wrath of god here, folks. James had to have known he couldn't exit the relationship quietly. That's like trying to leave a funeral with a tambourine tied to your shoe. He seemed upset at me when it didn't go according to plan.

When the exchange was finally over and the roaring of his engine had fallen into the distance, I dropped the bouncy ball and my head. I sat on the porch for an hour, digging through five years' worth of birthday cards, pictures, gifts, and notes. It was all there. All the love that had gone to waste. All this *shit*. And at the bottom of a dusty box was Berlitz. There he sat, blue and resolute. Next to him was the last letter I'd mailed James, the love questionnaire that was supposed to save our relationship.

It was unopened. For a solid minute I forgot to breathe. Then I ripped the letter up like a madwoman, making sure to annihilate every word on the pages. I took everything off the porch, walked it to the dumpster, and placed it next to last night's Chinese. But I clung to Berlitz, wondering how we'd ended up here in the first place.

As I cried on my porch with the last remnants of my grandfather in my quivering hands, I was vulnerable and strong, befuddled and clear. And for these moments of pain and heartache, I thank James for making me strong enough to overcome more than I ever imagined I could.

## What Doesn't Kill You Makes You Skinnier

Listen, I've got love handles. I've got jiggles. When I brush my teeth, my tummy quakes, and honestly I'm not entirely bummed about it. Because, you see, I love this thing called food. Salty food, sweet food, food covered in other food, food hidden inside other food—I love it all. Or I did, rather, before I got shit-canned in the love department.

The breakup took a toll on my body, and my appetite vanished. This was devastating for someone like me. I'd take a single bite of food and feel queasy enough to stop eating altogether. My roommates had to force-feed me. I lost ten pounds instantly.

I want to stop here for a second and confront something. I'd been a woman for twenty-two years, with my own inner dialogue about my figure. But I couldn't help being concerned about myself and this sudden weight loss. Part of me got excited. *Look at how skinny I am; he's going to rue the day he dumped me.* But mostly I tweaked out at the fact that I hadn't weighed this little since puberty. I knew deep down that I wasn't healthy. I knew I should have been giving my body more care and affection, not starving it out.

So what did I do? I tuned out all logic and began running like a crazy person. I'd always loved running, even when nobody was chasing me. Somehow I thought this could counterbalance my inability to eat. It didn't occur to me that I was wrecking myself even more.

The heartbreak pushed me over the edge. I signed up for the Bolder Boulder 10K and the Denver Rock 'n' Roll Half Marathon for the summer and fall. I was going to rebuild myself from the ground up. I was going to drink a lot of coffee and eat a cube of cheese if I felt like passing out. I was going to be skinnier than that trollop

James walked out on me for.

I ran the 10K within weeks of the breakup and sobbed the entire last mile. It was therapeutic and painful. This was not only the longest distance I'd ever run, but also the first time I felt like I wasn't counting on James to be there for me. I'd done this by myself. The only person who'd gotten me through the long runs in the blistering heat was me. Every step I took of that race was my own. The sunburn was entirely my doing.

After the 10K, I decided to push myself physically and began researching and training for the half marathon. I figured I wouldn't go full-blown marathon. I'd start with the half, then sign up for a full, then become the first female president. I printed out a twelve-week training guide and ran five times a week. I thought I was a total badass, and my legs looked awesome. Suck it, heartbreak.

Throughout the summer I continued to look thin. I lost my appetite indefinitely while working at the children's summer camp, where lunches consisted of PB&Js, hot dogs, and chicken fingers. These repulsed me and made me even less likely to feed myself. You just can't eat the same few items for an entire summer and feel okay about your life decisions. Plus, I had to be skinnier than my newest obsession, James's girlfriend, Molly the Trollop.

Worse was the lunch mess. Even the neatest small humans can't put food in their mouths correctly. One camper in particular I tried to avoid every day. *Timothy*. I would wait to sit down at lunch until he found a seat in the picnic area; then I'd choose a table as far away from him as possible. Sometimes I'd just pace the playground, keeping my eyes on him like a hawk from behind a pillar or plastic tray. But Timothy always found me. He'd squeeze in right next to me and dump seven packets of every condiment onto his hot dog and then miss his mouth completely as he shoveled a footlong at his tiny face.

"Timothy, you get *one* ketchup packet today." I turned my head for a millisecond.

"No, Timothy! Timothy, *no!*" I'd yell as he squirted mustard past his food and onto my arm. *Timothy, I swear to god, you were a mistake. You were an accident, Timothy. A giant, messy accident.*

Of course I didn't tell him he was an accident. But I really fucking wanted to. I tried to contain his mess, but to no avail. He always managed to cover his face and hair with some sort of sticky substance. Talk about gag reflex. I lost another ten pounds that summer sitting with Tim the Messy Accident Man Taylor.

The worst part about my receding waistline was that the country club where the camp was held had a scale in the women's locker room. This meant that every day I could see the number on the scale getting smaller. Maybe I'd always wanted to be thinner, but not like this. Never like this. Fucking James. Fucking Timothy.

This wasn't the body I was used to. I was transforming, and I was doing it by choice. It was like I had stepped into someone else's skin, where ribs could be seen through my shirts and the smell of ketchup made me vomit. The running may have added muscle tone to my legs, but I was still a mere shadow of who I'd once been.

I trudged through summer camp with massive amounts of coffee and running, thinking that my growing tiredness was nothing to be concerned about. I blamed this lack of energy on my thyroid disease, a blessing from both sides of my family genetically. I didn't think then that I was pushing myself to the breaking point. But it was getting worse. My coworkers started calling me out when I yawned while leading camp games with the kids. I also fell asleep on the pool deck with a clipboard on my face. That happened.

My roommates became concerned. On weekends, I would lie around or walk through the house aimlessly, looking for something to distract me. Sometimes I'd flip through old pictures of James and me and cry before deleting them. My roommates would cook a big breakfast on these weekends and we'd eat family-style around the table. Except I wouldn't eat.

"Just two big bites, Mimi," Gina would say.

"I can't. I'm going to throw up just looking at it."

Mel would nudge my skinny elbow. "Try the toast. Put some jam on it," she'd tell me.

This force-feeding routine continued for several weeks. It was a new kind of low. I felt like I'd accidentally hooked my heart to the back of the *Titanic*, then watched it slowly rip out my mushy soul as it sank and the onlookers waved as if nothing had happened. Forget bringing the lifeboats back around. Everyone was dead, and I just saw Rose kick Jack off the floating door.

It's no coincidence that it's called *heartache* and not *heart paper cut*. And I was surrounded by giggly children who mocked me with their carefree attitudes and affinity for Ring Pops. Sometimes they were so cute, it was hard to be angry at them, even when these tiny buffoons found love before I did. If I witnessed enough young love affairs, I was sure I was going to die alone. Therefore I needed to live vicariously through these kiddos and their ability to make love look like a breezy romantic comedy.

The opportunity arose one day with Jake and Millie[1], ages four and five. Millie was a regular at camp. She was involved in tennis, golf, and swim lessons, so I can hardly see how she had time for a relationship, but whatever. Jake was a newbie; he wasn't like the other boys at camp. He was sensitive. He hung out with the female counselors and didn't pick fights. He even hugged me once. I loved him. Millie caught his eye one day as I was holding him in his swimming towel like a tiny burrito.

He saw her from across the pool deck. She sauntered to her backpack to find her goggles. It was a hot day at camp, so we'd been trying to keep them in the water for

---

1.      Names have been changed to protect their marriage.

as long as possible, and we'd taken a break from the pool to move them to the field for water games. It was time to reapply sunscreen. We were on high alert, feeling kids' tiny faces for traces of oily sunscreen, as this was the only way to truly tell if they were deceiving us. Kids always lied about how much sunscreen they'd applied.

Jake gazed from me to Millie with big, adoring eyes. "I want Millie to use my special sunscreen," he said, like a true winner.

Some parents sent fancy and expensive sunscreens to camp with their children. Like everything else you leave in the charge of a small child, it almost always gets lost. Counselors were usually blamed for the irresponsibility of a kiddo who would lose their own head if it weren't attached to their shoulders. Jake handed Millie his twenty-dollar bottle of sunscreen, and she slathered it on her face and nose, quickly getting some in her eye and screaming bloody murder. I used my sleeve to wipe it out of her eyes. Jake stood nearby, looking worried for his woman.

We checked and doubled-checked for sunscreen, camp bracelets, water bottles, and towels, and wrangled the kids into line. Millie took her place as line leader, the most prestigious of camp careers. Jake hustled to stand beside her, in awe of her prowess.

"M-millie, you can use my towel if you want to," Jake said.

"Okay." Millie was unimpressed.

"Can I hold your hand?" Jake said with the valor of a thousand soldiers in battle.

"I guess so," Millie said, only slightly more impressed than before.

They held hands in line as we walked to the field. I was beside myself. I leaped over to my fellow female counselors and gossiped like a New Yorker at a hot dog stand.[2] Here was a boy who asked permission to hold a girl's hand. Why couldn't I find a boy like that? Who was my age? This camp romance was so innocent and genuine.

---

2.    I have no idea if New Yorkers gossip at hot dog stands. If you know anything about this, please feel free to send me hate mail.

Watching these small children play in ignorance of heartbreak was surreal. Someday they'd grow up—they'd graduate high school, pick careers, fall in and out of love. But for now they were just blurry little images on the playground, skinning their knees on rocks and soaring through the air on swings.

The first time is always the worst time. That's what *they* say, anyway. And they're probably right. I was young, naive, and determined to transform my body in hopes that I'd prove James wrong, that he'd regret walking away if he saw I was different. I was half-right; I did need to change, and in time I would. But I was still deep in my web, spinning my fantasy that my love for him could conquer everything, even my own broken head.

Instead of looking inside to fix the problem, I looked to the outside—to my body— to change. The weight came off faster and faster. I mutated into a new shape, hoping to become something that could be admired. I ran miles and miles and wore down my shoes, never stopping until I collapsed. I would break again, and soon—and this time the cleanup would be a hell of a lot worse.

Who smells a comeback story? I do. But only if it's not accompanied by ketchup or mayonnaise. Fuck that shit. *gags*

# Dating and Other Funny Shit

I consider myself an old soul. The fact that I became skilled at the art of wheelchair only confirms this. There may have been an error in the universe department, because I really should have been born a hundred years ago, making me young enough during the Great Depression to not give as much of a shit, but old enough to really hit my stride in my twenties during World War II. But also probably dead by now.

The 1940s was an era of classy women, brave soldiers, and true romance. The Greatest Generation not only battled in the trenches of Europe, but they also really knew how to date. When's the last time a guy asked your parents if he could court you, fought Nazis in your honor, kept your picture in his helmet, and wrote to you every day? Exactly.

My generation—the glued-to-the-screen, trend-recycling twenty-somethings of the world—has no conceptual understanding of relationships. We surround ourselves with apps that convince us we're more connected to each other than we actually are. We are the instant gratification generation that has lost touch of getting in touch with others. God forbid we lose our Wi-Fi connection too.

Unless you're cool and live in a cave somewhere, you and 99.9 percent of the rest of us submit to using technology in some way. And if I'm being 99.9 percent honest, most of my friends found out about my brain hemorrhage via Snapchat. But that's not the point. These things can only add to our quality of life; they cannot *become* our lives. And during my rock-bottom post-James summer, technology became my main tool of self-destruction as I spiraled out of sanity watching his romance blossom with another woman.

Then I found dating apps.

I'm going to let you in on a little secret because most people don't know this. And because I like you. The popular hookup app Tinder was invented long ago, at the height of the post-plague European witch trials. Kings and lords and archbishops would scour the land for beautiful women to carry on their line of descent. Can archbishops carry on a line of descent? Okay, the kings and lords and *possibly* archbishops would gather together the most beautiful women from across the land.

Once the women were in the castle, they were lined up and examined using a complex scale that ranked women based on facial features, waist measurements, and credit score. If a woman was considered desirable, the king would whisk his hand to the right, and they would be taken to his chambers for late-night pleasures. If the king swiped his hand to the left, the women were deemed witches and burned. As tinder for the fire. Too soon?

When James displayed his new love journey all over social media, I took that as my cue to find my own new Prince Charming. If he could move on quickly, then by golly, so could I! This is when I became a tad promiscuous. Calm down, Mom. I didn't do anything stupid. I just went on a lot of bad dates. And some good ones. Shall we begin?

First on the list: Creepy Face-Holding Guy. Why yes, yes, it was as terrifying as it sounds.

I was sitting on my friend Lexi's couch, brooding as I pulled up Molly's Instagram. *Who does she think she is, that trollop,* I thought. *She probably isn't even funny. I bet her laugh sounds stupid.*

"Would you knock that off?" Lexi called from the kitchen. This was my eighth sadness-induced social media episode in three days, and her patience with me was dwindling. "For Christ's sake, Mimi," she said. "Just get the Tinder app."

After a few minutes of testing the swipe feature, I right-swiped a guy who had similarly found my face attractive. We started talking, and within twenty-four hours I had agreed to meet him at Chautauqua Park in Boulder for a morning hike and some tea. Harmless, right? *Wrong.*

This was the first date I had been on since James, and I was a chump. I told no one where I was going. Strike one. I met the new guy early in the morning in an obscure location. Strike two.

A vague compact car pulled into the dirt parking lot at 6:03 a.m. He got out of his car and we greeted, if you could call it that. It wasn't awkward in the "do we shake hands or hug?" kind of way. It was awkward because he held my face. You read that right. *He held my face and stared directly into my eyeballs.* I mean, I've heard I have the bluest eyes west of the Mississippi, but come on, guy.

I detached myself from his hands and made a snap decision not to kick him in the shins and run away screaming. So he was a little touchy. No big deal.

He unloaded several large bins full of Mason jars and a miniature French press, then opened each jar of "herbs" and asked me to sniff them. I complied as he rambled off complicated names of plants which I questioned the legality of. He made a concoction of said possibly-contraband and put it in the French press.

"Thankkkkk youuuuuu," I said with heavy suspicion as he handed me a cup of freshly brewed mystery.

He rolled a joint as I contemplated my next move, which was to follow him up the mountain, obviously. I claim complete responsibility for my stupid decisions; I was born with an overwhelmingly dangerous trust in other people. This is why every old-school Disney princess in the history of all time let the guy save her instead of demanding a background check. Quite frankly, I'm pleasantly surprised I haven't been kidnapped by an axe murderer yet. If you're an axe murderer and you're reading this, I bet you can find my home address in this book somewhere. I trust you, though.

I followed Creepy Face-Holding Guy up the mountain, presumably to my death. As we walked, his hands wandered to my waist. I pushed him away and extended my distance to a radius of ten feet. He tried again for my hand. *Nope, sorry, dude— I've got a radius to uphold.* At one point I was so far away that I was shouting my responses to his small talk.

We reached a fence post and sat. I was strict on the ten-foot policy. He continued to smoke his herbs and discuss at length his knowledge of the fifth dimension. *This is the strangest human I have ever seen*, I thought. *Why did I agree to this?*

"You're so far away," he said as I squirmed back from him again.

At this point I told him the truth: I had just gotten out of a serious relationship and wasn't ready for this sort of thing. I omitted the fact that I was totally wigged out by the touchiness and didn't want to be made into a lampshade that day. I went for the "you seem like a really nice guy" approach instead. He was pissed.

"Well, maybe you shouldn't waste people's time!" he said. He threw his cup of tea on the ground and stormed off the mountain. I looked around to see if anyone else was on hand to witness this epic fail, and when I realized I was alone, I gave myself a slow clap.

This somehow did not deter me from continuing my Tinder search for Prince Charming. Some weeks later I booked a new sketchy adventure, further proving my ability to put myself in ridiculously dangerous situations. Again, Mom, I'm sorry.

After texting for a few days, we decided to meet. After midnight. I picked him up from his house and drove us to a park near my place. I didn't tell anyone where I was going. Mind you, I truly believed this to be innocent at the time. Even Snow White was fooled by that shiny apple. She was a vegan. She needed natural sugars.

Walk in the Park Guy and I enjoyed an hour of climbing trees and talking about Disney musicals. We walked around the park and played on the jungle gym. I thought he was perfect. He craved more heroines like Mulan. He liked improv and had an adult job. He checked all my tiny boxes. He took my glasses off sweetly, putting them in his pocket to keep them safe, and kissed me on the sidewalk. Maybe I'd found him, my new prince.

After a few hours of holding hands in the park, I drove him back to his house to call it a night. But he wanted to hang out with me even more.

"Want to sit on my hammock and watch the stars?" he said.

We kissed and cuddled in the hammock, and I started to think this Tinder business was the real deal.

"Why don't you come in and watch a movie or something?"

I thought this a fine idea too. I was a doe-eyed damsel; I didn't really understand what he meant. Cut me some slack, will ya? I hadn't been in the dating game since I was seventeen. Ladies: watching a movie does not actually mean watching a movie. I mean, if you're talking to me, it does. I take my movie watching very seriously.

So I agreed. I loved cuddling, and I loved critiquing the cinematography of popular movies. How could I refuse? Then he started getting strange. His kisses became more forceful, and we moved to his room. I realized he wasn't going to put *Forrest Gump* on after all.

"Hey, what you think is going to happen is not going to happen," I said. "Can't we just watch a movie like you said?"

When I stopped his advances, he *moped*. He sulked because I didn't want to have sex with him. I felt like I was at summer camp in a standoff with a seven-year-old over why he couldn't have a cookie for lunch. I lay on the bed in shock. He slumped over and mumbled angrily. I thought that maybe he'd snap out of it and we'd resume our conversation on Disney musicals or at least turn on *Forrest Gump* or something. He did not, and around six in the morning he had to go to work and walked me out the door.

Despite the awkward overnight interaction, I hoped he would call me. I'd like to use the excuse that my cognitive abilities were deranged, but at this point in the story they were textbook.

Next I met Nurse Tim. He was the only man I found on Tinder who didn't try to de-pants me the minute I met him. We had intellectual texting conversations with accurate grammar for a few weeks before we met in person. He spoke of feminism, his yoga practice, and the many interesting people he met working on the psych floor of a hospital. For our first date, he took me to a park by his house, but in the daylight this time. He laid out a picnic blanket and impressed me with his knowledge of wine that didn't come out of a box. He also brought chocolate chips. This Prince didn't appear to be a frog. I knew this because frogs didn't eat chocolate.

We went on more dates, but I began to distance myself. He would be sweet and try to kiss me, and I would slink backward or giggle. He'd call me on the phone at night, take me out to meet his friends. I told him that things were happening so fast. Here was a real Prince Charming, and I couldn't take it seriously. The wound in my heart was still open and gushing with goo. I wasn't ready for the real fairy tale.

After deciding on friendship with Nurse Tim, I convinced myself that he simply hadn't been the perfect prince for me. I carried on matching with complete strangers over the internet.

Part of me got excitement out of being reckless and single for the first time. But what I was doing was not healthy for my heart or my ticking time bomb of a brain. I was trying to rebound, follow reflex; do *something*. What I should have been doing was focusing on my needs, something I hadn't done for a long time. I'm positive my mother wasn't a fan of the behavior either.

Nevertheless, Secret Agent Man happened. We met for a first date at a hipsteresque restaurant, and he bought me appetizers. His eyes were a fun chocolaty brown that reminded me of James. When he spoke, it was like he was whispering secrets that I wanted to know. We talked for a few hours and then strolled around in the fancy part of downtown. That was an upgrade from dark parks and stained couches. He insisted that I walk on the inside of the sidewalk, something I understood to be an act of gentlemanliness. Prince Charming school had taught him well.

Our first kiss happened on the second date. We continued to walk around parks and drink coffee, which gave me plenty of opportunity to make a fool of myself. I wore heels on one date and had to take them off because my feet hurt so badly. But what did I say to explain this behavior?

"Sorry, I need to air out my feet," I told him. "Because they smell." What the hell was that about? Perhaps I wasn't born with the smooth gene.

A few weeks into our affair, he became weird and shady. We'd have an amazing date; then he wouldn't talk to me for three days. I tried to play it cool. I said I was busy anyway. Let's be honest, I was staring at my phone all day long, waiting for him to reappear like my long-lost Christmas socks.

I'm not one to play games. If I like you, I'm going to tell you about it. I bake a lot of banana bread for male suitors, and it sometimes freaks them out. But that's my style. The go-to behavior in dating culture these days is to go back and forth like a pinball machine until one party reluctantly "catches feelings." I was never good at pinball machines in the first place, and I'm especially sucky at this one. Plus, I like baking too much.

This on-again, off-again limbo continued for several weeks, and it drove me insane. He was a private investigator, which to my understanding was like any investigator on TV who had to go to strip clubs to find bad guys. He was very secretive about his job, though, I guess for obvious reasons. He had a badge and sometimes carried a gun. I was very, very into this. He was like a superhero. A prince with superpowers and tighter clothing.

I'm no Halle Berry, okay? I don't emerge from glistening pools of water looking sexy. I scared away Bond, James Bond by inviting him to be my date at my roommate's wedding. Maybe he only heard *my* and *wedding* and decided he wasn't ready to put a ring on it. But why wouldn't you want to be my date at a festival of love where you get to drink tons of (usually) free alcohol and dance like a maniac? Even if it's not my fairy tale, it's still cute as shit.

After I asked him to accompany me to the wedding, he disappeared, never to be seen or heard from again. I guess he must be a pretty good secret agent. Or Goldfinger finally caught up with him and is interrogating him in a dark basement as we speak.

There were other guys that summer, a few of whom were put on the chopping block during revisions of this book. Which sounds horrific, but I assure you, it was pretty painless. For me, anyway. There were good dates, bad dates, and a teacher who bought me cheese fries so delicious that I considered proposing to him on the first date. I wasn't a crazy person, okay? I just liked cheese fries. All right, I was a little messed up. It's almost like I was asking for a head injury to snap me out of my cheesy delusions.

Last on the love failure list—at least for a long while—was Day of Brain Hemorrhage Guy. Now, I didn't know Day of Brain Hemorrhage Guy was Day of Brain Hemorrhage Guy until several months later, but I thought it was a good way of naming him. You'll see.

We agreed on a bar in Denver with live music and draft brews. I was less than a week away from my first day of school as a student teacher and was reeling with anxiety and half-baked lesson plans. My car had also broken down earlier in the week, which was comical, considering the shit that's about to go down in a second.

My parents brought me to the school in the morning, and my mentor, Lindsay, dropped me off at the bar for the date. It was a team effort getting me to Day of Brain Hemorrhage Guy.

When he arrived, I quickly saved my work—I'd pulled out my laptop to complete my first day of school PowerPoint—and threw my computer into my bag. I felt a tiny surge of pressure in my head. *Great, I'm so stressed, I've given myself a headache,* I thought.

"Hi, I'm Mimi, how are you?" I said.

"I'm Day of Brain Hemorrhage Guy, fine, thank you," he said.

Okay, so he didn't say that. But I honestly can't remember his name.

We ordered some appetizers (geez, what *is* it with me and appetizers?) and made small talk. I chugged a beer, hoping the alcohol could get me through both the headache and the mediocre date. Something was off. He seemed like a nice guy; I just didn't think we had anything in common. In hindsight, it was probably equal parts brain bleed and him being kind of uninteresting.

We parted ways for the evening, and I called my parents to come pick me up from the bar.

"How'd it go?" Mom asked from the front seat.

"The meetings were so long today, and the date was boring," I said. "And now my car is broken, and I'm not going to be able to get to school, and I don't have any money, and…" I spiraled into an emotional fit and began sobbing in the backseat.

Dad gave Mom a worried glance. "Goodness, sweetheart, it's going to be just fine!"

They must have thought it was a bit dramatic to be sobbing about a bland date, a few meetings, and a routine trip to the auto body shop. And indeed it was. Because deep inside my cerebellum there'd been a tiny explosion; at that very moment, a pool of blood was growing inside my brain.

Day of Brain Hemorrhage Guy, if you're reading this, I'm sorry I didn't text you back—my brain was kind of hemorrhaging. But that's a story for a second date.

## Teacher for a Day

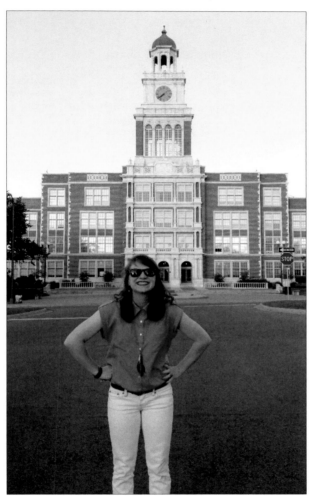

*Proudly showing off my school pre–brain burst.*

I lasted one week, actually. Okay, five days. To be fair, I taught for 685 minutes. This is only 11.416 hours. It took me a long time to dig up the old bell schedule and figure that out (round of applause).

This total does not account for the thirty-some hours of training and meetings that occurred the week prior to students showing up to my class without a pencil for the first and certainly not the last time. I was at the beginning of my journey, ready to check off my Sassy Career Woman box. Student teaching would get me a teaching license, and getting a teaching license would bring me one step closer to having my own classroom.

I'd been excited to start this journey long before James left the picture, but now it felt even more important to be teaching for real. To me, the classroom meant adulthood. It meant stable ground after the uncertainty of the past few months. Putting on my pencil skirt and dusting off my ready-made lesson plans from my college courses gave me new optimism and strength.

I thought I had prepared my entire life to be a teacher. Safe in my mother's photo album is a picture of my cousin Kayla and me in matching dresses, sitting atop my aunt Karen's towering teacher chair, from back when we'd help her organize her classroom in the summertime. I'd spend hours at her cluttered desk, wrapping rubber bands around sets of colored pens. I'd disinfect each desk and re-center every inspirational poster. Aunt Karen and I would take trips to the craft store to pick out new borders for her bulletin boards and grab cheeseburgers on the way back to school. I had to stand on chairs to staple the fabric to the wall, squinting one eye and moving my head back and forth to see if it was level. I still squint sometimes to make sure there is only one of something instead of two. That's pretty normal for my head injury, though.

In my imaginary classroom, I'd have all my sharpened pencils in clean cups. I would separate piles of graded and to-be-graded papers with polka-dotted binder clips. By the end of each day, the bright sticky note marking the to-be-graded pile could be recycled, because I'd always be timely in giving my students feedback. I would also be great about saving the planet and would hardly ever have to make copies. Every poster would be centered on my immaculate walls, and my students' smiles would match my brightly colored bulletin boards.

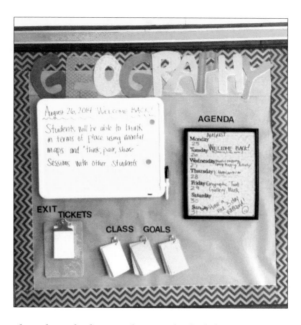

*Day one, a.k.a. the only day my shit ever looked this nice in my classroom.*

I have a lot of teachers in my family, going all the way back to my great-grandmother Bertha, who had a one-room schoolhouse at the age of eighteen in Keota, Iowa. She taught a student who would someday become Grandpa Glessy. It's also rumored that he might not have been a student at all, but the window washer. I didn't plan on following in Bertha's footsteps and marrying one of my students/window washers, but the idea of a one-room schoolhouse delighted me.

In my final semester at CU Boulder, I began planning for my student teaching semester. The university claimed no responsibility for securing this assignment, so it was up to me, amid a downwardly spiraling relationship with James, to find a place to teach. I squeezed meetings with teachers and principals in between my history classes and sat in traffic daydreaming about my imaginary schoolhouse. It didn't exist outside my mind, and it would never exist if I couldn't find a teacher who trusted me—a stranger—to teach their very real students.

Then I rolled down City Park Esplanade at ten o'clock one warm morning in April, just a month before graduation. I'd been down this street many times before with James. We enjoyed going to the record store across the street to find new music and frequented the Chipotle and the Tattered Cover Book Store next door. I'd never really looked across to the other side at the towering castle before me.

Now I paused at the stop sign and gawked at the building as several kids crossed. The building stood four stories tall, billowing up from the ground like an institution of hope and promise. The windows glistened, nearly blinding me as a car behind me honked for me to move forward. I pulled into the parking lot and rushed to the sidewalk for a closer look. Trees lined the campus, and the front doors were centered perfectly on three marble pillars. The bulk of the building towered up to an old green clock that ticked ever so slightly. It was Hogwarts. I was looking upon Cinderella's castle itself. I'd found my muse: East High School.

I met with a history and geography teacher named Lindsay Anderson to discuss the possibility of me joining her in the fall. When I watched Lindsay teach, I was mesmerized. She was quirky and sweet, kind and respected. The kids loved her. It wasn't hard for me to fall in love with her too. I sat at a tiny desk while the students asked questions and engaged. She told them stories and kept them on task. They waved her goodbye as they exited the room.

"What do you think?" she asked that afternoon.

"I think this looks amazing!" I nearly shouted. I would have given a limb to work with her. And I guess I sort of did. Or do you consider the brain a limb?

The idea that I could remotely compare to a teacher like Lindsay was a fantasy. I'd gone through teaching school. I'd

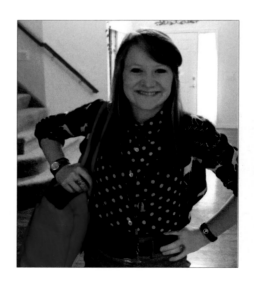

written lesson plans and taught random groups of teenagers in classrooms across the Denver metro. But it was all in a vacuum. The lessons weren't kid-proof. In theory, they would be amazing—if I had a classroom of robots with no socioeconomic struggles or problems with their robot parents. When I taught classes, they'd been under the watchful eye of the real teacher, the one who could make the kids suffer real consequences if they didn't behave themselves during my corny and "engaging" lesson on World War II fighter pilots. Lindsay was the teacher I wanted to be when I grew out of my fantastical immaturity.

Lindsay agreed to take me on as her student teacher for the fall of 2014. I would teach three sections of ninth grade honors geography. I was excited at the prospect of a younger grade because I lack authority, looking like a ninth-grader myself. I naively assumed they would respect me despite our small age difference. I was also excited to study geography for the first time since high school.

Going into secondary education with an emphasis in social studies meant that I had to know everything in the entire universe: history, sociology, psychology, economics, geography, civics, and astronomy. That's why teachers make the big bucks. But I didn't know much about geography other than what I'd failed twice before finally passing the teacher licensure exam. I would have to pretend. It wouldn't be lying, exactly, just playing make-believe. I was good at that.

I bought a bright red laptop bag and filled it to the brim with binder clips and fancy folders, which I'd need to organize my fantastic lesson plans and impeccable student work. I got ready early in the morning and packed my lunch for the first day.

Mom came down the stairs at six o'clock in her robe, her hair half in curlers. "First day picture!" she said as she danced around the kitchen.

"Come on, Mom, really?"

"We'll make it a tradition! Go stand by the door."

I complied and smiled through my terror. Then I got in my car and drove to school with my hands tightly gripping the hot leather wheel.

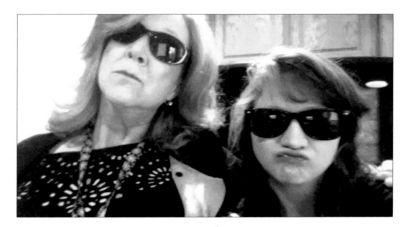

*We're badass. We know.*

I arrived at East High and walked in the front doors, clinging to the sound of slamming lockers and rustling backpacks. I was doing it. I was a teacher. Kind of. I wouldn't be teaching a class until fourth period, leaving me just enough time to make five pots of coffee and panic my face off.

By the time a gaggle of students had entered the classroom for my first geography class of the day, I was exhausted, but I thought that if I chugged a few more cups of coffee, maybe nobody would notice. Now it was showtime.

"Welcome, everyone! My name is Ms. Hayes! Find a seat anywhere you like for today, and we'll get started!" My smile was plastered so forcefully to my face, I must have looked like a psychotic clown.

The kids rummaged around their empty bags for pencils. Some greeted new friends they had made last period. They were gangly and quiet, yet to reveal personalities and quirks. Their cell phones stuck out of their pockets as they shifted in their chairs during my painfully long explanation of who I was and why I was there.

"I will be your student teacher for this semester," I said. "I'm a student at the University of Colorado Boulder. After this semester, I will receive my teaching license. Mrs. Anderson is my teaching mentor—she works here at East High School, and I am taking over her geography classes."

Their expressions ranged from "not enthused" to "how old is she *really*?"

After I'd mispronounced even the simplest of names on the attendance roster, we moved on to our first activity: creating mental maps of the world *sans* textbooks.

"We can't use our phones either?" a student whose name I couldn't pronounce blurted out.

"They're called mental maps," I said. "We have to use our brains and our brains only." A lot of good my brain would do me here. At this point I was becoming a leaky faucet.

They sighed in unison and grouped up around the room. I handed out giant rolls of butcher paper and noticed they were heavier than I'd expected them to be.

"Your job is to create a map of the world using just the images in your head. If you're not sure, take your best guess. There are no penalties for trying!"

"Can we use scissors?"

"No can do! You need to rip the paper into the shapes of the continents as best you can."

I immediately got death glares. "Miss, it's going to be all messy!"

"Learning is messy!" I said, feeling like Hilary Swank in *Freedom Writers*. Ironically, I'd been spilling coffee all over myself for the past few hours, leaving stains on my skirt. My eyelids were heavy with exhaustion. *Must be all this learning we're doing*, I thought. Wrong.

When they were done, we toured the room to view their maps. The students knew what North America looked like and had placed it in the top left corner.

"That map is *weird*," one student said.

"To us, yes, it does look strange. But it all depends on who's looking at it. This week we're going to be talking about ethnocentrism. Let's write that in our notebooks, *eth-no-cen-trism*, very good…"

I didn't make it to ethnocentrism. At least not then, anyway. I collected one written assignment, several permission slips, and approximately forty signed syllabi. I took notes while Lindsay taught her juniors and seniors. I attended the first staff meeting of the year and wrote "Student Learning Outcomes" in bright blue ink at the top of my notebook, with a gigantic question mark beside it. I timed my lessons down to the minute, then realized that teaching was unpredictable, and it didn't matter that I'd allowed five minutes to wrap up this activity, because there's a fire drill today and I'd be putting out bigger fires in my own body soon enough.

I started to get sick as my first week went on. I was off-balance and queasy and had to cling to Lindsay to get through the crowded hallways. It was strange and unsettling and frustrating. My first week out of the real adulthood gate, and the universe was already fucking with me. Hadn't I been screwed enough? I wanted so badly for this job to distract me from my James turmoil and set me free.

On Wednesday I leaned over to pick up a pencil and immediately saw stars. I stumbled over myself during class. In between classes on Thursday I went to the bathroom and almost fell onto the floor when I bent to squat above the toilet. *That's odd*, I thought. *I'm not normally this clumsy, am I?*

"Didn't you go to urgent care last weekend?" Lindsay asked over lunch.

"Yeah." I bit into my sandwich. Because I hadn't lost an arm to a joust, my condition had not appeared serious enough for urgent care to suggest further medical attention. They'd given me some Dramamine, which obviously wasn't working. "I'm going to see my doctor Friday," I said. "Maybe she'll give me something else."

I sought a magic pill, a wave of a wand, something mystical to bring me out of my dizzy misery. I'd been suspecting an ear infection—I'd read somewhere that when your ears were messed up, you'd run into walls and shit. I knew nothing about my inner ear, but I knew it was pounding and that this was a problem.

I took home my first binder-clipped to-be-graded assignments that weekend. *These will be done in no time*, I thought as I perched atop Mom's kitchen counter with a cup of tea. But when I sat down to grade them, my stomach lurched. Maybe their grammar was so bad, it was making me sick. Maybe it was this hieroglyphic writing I had to decipher. I got queasy looking down at the papers, so I held them above my face at an upward angle.

Mom raised her eyebrows at me. "What are you doing there, sweet pea?"

"Just trying to read this kid's writing," I said. "I think it's in code."

I riffled through my stacks to count my permission slips. As part of my licensure program, I was required to evaluate my own practice and turn in a summative assessment, including student work samples, commentary from colleagues, and videos of my teaching, which I needed parent permission for.

I'd handed out the permission slips on the first day and made extra copies for the students who would cram it in their bags, never to be seen again. I was still short twenty permission slips. I copied their names down in my little blue notebook and marked the page with a sticky note: "Ask for permission slips!"

The assessment portfolio was due mid-October, a mere month and a half after school started. I was overwhelmed already. The portfolio required answering fifty essay questions with evidence of my students' proficiency in essential content. I also needed ten unedited minutes of teaching perfection, but I needed to get to know my students first and get a handle on teaching for the first time. I needed to pronounce their names correctly on film. I needed everyone to please raise their hands and speak clearly into this high-definition microphone. I needed to stop tripping over Cody's skateboard. And I needed all those damn permission slips.

I could feel October 16 crashing in on me. It turned out that this date would have a different significance; my brain had other plans for me. I just didn't know it yet.

## Mother Knows Best

*My mom, super relaxed and hanging with some Teletubbies
after I nearly killed her with a 10K.*

Every fairy tale needs a good queen. She's strong and respected and can determine the fate of your pathetic farm while simultaneously keeping the country out of war and beheading adversaries in her spare time. She's intense as *fuck*.

It's no surprise that I grew up to be a badass. I come from a long line of female goddesses, and my mother is no exception to the lineage. She'll get you to clean your damn room and will whip your local Girl Scout troop into shape while she balances five side hustles you didn't even know about. She is constantly putting my needs above her own. Anytime I have fallen sick, my mother has known about it before I did.

"Of course you feel tired," she'll say. "It's all the UV rays. Eat more paprika. It blocks free radicals." It's a Mom thing.

She got pretty heavy on the Mom thing when I showed my initial symptoms the first week of school.

Our first urgent care visit a few days before I began student teaching had ended with us being rushed out of the examination room by a grumpy nurse who brushed off my symptoms as vertigo and handed me a bottle of Dramamine. My next step was to meet with Dr. Pollock under Mom's watchful eye.

Mom had suggested weeks prior to make an appointment about my extreme fatigue, something I'd battled throughout the summer. She suspected an imbalance with my thyroid. "You probably need a new dosage of meds," she said. I was tired as ever from teaching for the first time, but now the dizziness and throbbing ears were starting to weird me out. I'd had an underactive thyroid gland since age twelve; maybe all this James shit was catching up to me too. Maybe the doctor would tell me I'd picked up some strange heartbreak disease (I hoped to god it wasn't an STD).

I told the doctor that the Dramamine wasn't working. I was getting worse. I'd become a clumsy mess, tripping off curbs and sidewalks or into my students' desks. I'd just met the kids. They probably thought I was drunk. I wasn't sure what Mom made of all that, but I know she was not about to handle what came out of Dr. Pollock's mouth next.

"These things happen," Dr. P said. "You're probably just tired. Have you dealt with depression before?"

My eyes began to roll back in my head. *Passing out, we're passing out! GOING DOWN*, I thought, and I rested my head on the paper-covered examination table and lost consciousness.

"Hello? She just passed out," my mother was saying as a nurse cracked a can of orange juice in front of my nose, bringing me to my senses. "She isn't depressed. She's sick!"

This didn't seem to concern Dr. Pollock too much. Maybe people passed out on her examination table all the time. Maybe her patients cried wolf and made a big deal out of a paper cut. Hey, "these things happen."

We went home, and I continued at full speed while Mom invented reasons for why I was feeling so weird. I had volunteered for another season at the murder mystery theater in Gold Hill, Colorado, and was cast in a show for Saturday, August 30. I'd started the previous summer with the troupe. This year the theme was time travel and the trends of the 1870s and 1970s. If there's one thing I love more than fairy tales, it's time travel murder mysteries. I played a snobby rich daughter and had a killer white lace pantsuit.

But I began complaining about my real-life health in the dressing room. "I don't feel like myself," I told them. "I'm clumsy lately."

The show lasted two and a half hours, with dinner for the guests served in between. We mingled with the guests as they tried to identify which of us was the murderer. While I appeared to be stumbling and suspicious, it was not I who murdered Dr. Marmot in the salon with the time sphere. The cast kept an eye on me throughout the show so that I didn't tumble down any stairs.

"Maybe it's the altitude that's making you sick," Maggie said as she stroked my shaggy '70s wig. "You haven't been up for a show since last season."

When I returned from the mountains, I was happy to have Labor Day to relax before returning to teach on Tuesday. But even the long weekend couldn't cure the now nonstop throbbing in my ears. Mom tucked Dr. Pollock's business card in my wallet and told me to call her office again as soon as it opened.

On Tuesday morning I convinced myself that I would power through the pain. I grabbed a banana and some green tea for breakfast and headed out the door to my now fixed PT Cruiser. As I drove, I took a bite of the banana and sipped my tea. My stomach lurched. The princess was going to throw up in her own carriage.

I quickly pulled over at a gas station just blocks from my house and threw open the car door, not bothering to grab my phone or lock the car behind me. I staggered inside the dingy bathroom. I knelt in my heels and pencil skirt and coughed up the bite of banana and sip of tea and consciously broke my one golden rule: do not touch the toilet seat. Then I stood up, smoothed out my skirt, and went back to the car to call Lindsay.

"I just threw up," I said. "I must have had a bad banana. I don't think I should come in today."

Lindsay told me to stay home and that she would teach my classes until I returned healthy. When I got home from the gas station, I abandoned the rotting banana on the counter and moved directly to the nearest toilet. For the rest of the day, I lay in my bed with a trash bag huddled at my side.

Wednesday came, and my condition hadn't improved. I called in again to Lindsay, who was starting to get weirded out at yet another unidentified symptom. I was also concerned about all the puking. She ordered me to stay home for as many days as I needed. I emailed her the lessons I'd planned on teaching.

Because my mother is the Khaleesi of all the land, the breaker of chains, and the mother of three really weird kids, she decided to take matters into her own hands. She went to work and chatted up her co-worker's sister's cousin, who was a doctor. This doc recommended an inversion table, a giant torture-looking device meant to realign your back, to resettle the fluid behind my ears. They also suggested other exercises, like throwing my head against a pillow at Mach 1. Lo and behold, my parents already had an inversion table for Dad's cranky ol' back! Queen Mom was working her own magic and finding makeshift solutions to save the day.

That day, my older sister Erin strapped me in and flipped me upside down every half hour. We rotated back slowly, my head pounding while my stomach did acrobatics. I felt like an astronaut on a rocket ship ready to launch. *Projectile vomiting in T-minus ten, nine…*

We flipped upside down several times, rocking back and forth until I turned green. I carefully crawled into my parents' bed. Erin would report back to me in thirty minutes to repeat the process. Meanwhile, I lay in bed in agony while my stomach whirled from the reverse gravity experiment. I tried to take tiny sips of water and lie still. But then a few minutes into my statue game, I moved my head just a little to look at the clock. I rushed to the bathroom and vomited. I returned to the bed with a trash can.

*Don't move. You are a statue now.* But I needed a sip of water. I turned my eyes to the table while keeping my head still. I couldn't see the water, but I was determined. Maybe I could just move my head one degree to the left? *Nope.* Nausea overcame me, and I collapsed my entire face into the trash can, heaving into it and choking on my own spit and bile. I couldn't wait the half hour until Erin would pay me a visit. Maybe I'd be dead by then. I feebly reached around the bed for my cell phone and called her from upstairs.

"Something's not right," I moaned.

This was our first trip to the emergency room.

They called me into the examination room, hooked me up to machines, and prodded me with needles. They didn't say much about the purpose of the machines or needles, but I was told I was dehydrated. No shit. Erin and I waited for our parents to show up. We took the opportunity to make jokes.

"Which one of these plugs do you think is keeping you alive?" she asked.

"The big red one," I said. "Pull it and see what happens." I looked down at the plastic heart monitor clamped down on my right index finger. It was glowing red. I shakily pointed it at her nose. "I'll be riiiiiiiight heeeeere," I said in the most spot-on E.T. accent imaginable, and winced as my head jerked and the dizzy kicked in.

A few minutes later our parents erupted through the floorboards of the cramped room. A man came into the room with them and introduced himself as Nurse So-and-So.

"Let's take a look," he said, and pulled out a tiny flashlight to examine my ears. "Yep, you're all plugged up in there."

"Plugged up?" Mom said.

"There's some fluid behind your ears causing the pain. Make an appointment with an ear specialist."

Landing an appointment with a specialist would take months. I'd probably be dead by then. I giggled at my mom's four eyes. Everything else was double too. I didn't remember crossing my eyes.

"Mom, when did you grow two more eyes?" I asked as another nurse jabbed an IV in my arm.

Mom raised her four eyebrows at me. I let my gaze wander the room and wondered what portal I'd stumbled into that allowed me to see the world in this way. I tried focusing on my right shoe. Maybe if I focused hard enough, I could multiply it even more.

As I sat playing mind games about which hospital item I'd levitate, I felt dampness around me. The bed was soaking wet. The nurse accused me of wetting the bed, and it took all my nonexistent energy not to haul off and hit her. *I think I would know if I pissed myself, lady.*

Mom was pointing. "Her IV moved out of her arm. The entire bag is empty."

Nurse Rudeface left, annoyed, to get a new bag of salt water.

"It's not my fault she sucks at putting IVs in," I said to Mom's four eyes. "Some people's children. Wet the bed? I'd like to see her multiply things with her eyes!"

Mom's face changed. It was clear something was wrong with me, and she couldn't do a thing about it. The nurses determined that my ailment wasn't life-threatening and suggested making another appointment. Erin put my wet clothes in a bag, and I walked out of the emergency room in paper pants.

Mom's kingdom was disturbed. The entire car ride home, she steamed with anger and worry. Being a queen is hard. I can't imagine having a child birthed from your hoo-ha and watching it grow into a functioning human creature, only to have zero control when it grows up and runs into traffic or develops a rare and exotic brain thing. That sounds like the absolute worst.

The first ER visit had turned up inconclusive, and Mom wasn't satisfied. She instructed me to call my doctor to figure out what was going on. I sat in bed the next day, nauseous and spinny and cursing my inability to be with my students. I tried to contact my doctor. For five hours. Each time, I reached a nurse who reassured me that my doctor would call me back. Eventually.

Because we'd been told it was vertigo or some mutated ear infection, Mom advised me to follow up with the specialist that the ER nurse had suggested.

I punched in the number as I tried to make the two TV sets into four with my eyes. *Multiply. Multiply, damn you!* No luck. Not on the TV sets and not on the appointment. The receptionist on the other end informed me that I'd need a referral from my primary care doctor. You know, the one who was giving me the cold shoulder right now. I hung up the phone and called my mother.

"Dr. Pollock isn't going to do anything, Mom," I cried. "It's fine. I'll just go back to bed."

"Absolutely unacceptable," she said. "I'm coming home right now."

In what felt like milliseconds my mother burst through the door and whisked me into the car to take me back to the emergency room. My condition wasn't improving, and Mom was not going to settle for an appointment in five months. She wanted answers and she wanted them now.

As we opened the garage door, my phone rang. It was Dr. P.

"Oh, hi," I said with disgust. "My mother and I were just discussing when you'd call me back. We're going to the emergency room right—"

"Let me talk to her!" Mom shouted, and snagged the phone from my feeble hands.

"No, you listen right now," she fumed into the phone. "We're not going to wait. This is ridiculous. We're on our way to the ER."

"I think you're overreacting, Janet." Was the phone on speaker? "You need to fill a prescription of Valium and send her to bed," said Dr. P.

"You know what? Why don't you take that prescription and shove it up your ass!"

It's debated to this day if these were the last words my mother said to my doctor. Mom swears she was politer. There's no way of knowing, because she was going apeshit and my brain was all kinds of messed up. We'll just have to speculate.

When we got to the emergency room, this time at Saint Joseph Hospital, a nurse took my blood pressure and informed me that I was not dying, so it wasn't an emergency. My mom became Mega Mom. We waited for a room to meet with another nurse.

"What seems to be the problem?" the new nurse said.

"I don't know!" Mom was steaming again. "Why don't *you* tell me? We were just in the emergency room yesterday, and nobody seems to be worried that she's puking her guts out every time she moves her head."

The nurse put her finger in front of my face. "Do you see double?"

"No," I said.

"Looks normal," she said.

"No!" Mom sprang from her chair. "Look at this." She pushed the nurse aside and put her finger in front of my face, then moved the finger slowly to the left as my eyes followed. Everything doubled. "Does *this* look normal to you?"

If my eyes moved, everything became double. That was the trick. Shifting the eyes. I'd been going about it *all wrong.*

According to outside sources, if you looked at my eyes while they were following the finger to the left, you'd have thought I was experiencing an exorcism.

"We have spoken with our attorney," Mom said to Nurse Lazy-Finger. "We will do anything necessary to find out what is going on with our daughter." Damn, Mom. I didn't even know we had an attorney.

"I suppose an MRI wouldn't hurt," she said. "But you'll have to wait."

"We'll wait." Mom crossed her arms in defiance. It was like a scene straight outta *Game of Thrones.* The Mother of Dragons was awake. And she was pissed.

### Shit, Maybe I'm Not Okay

Do you remember the prologue? That first page you turned to way back when, the one that made you go all "Wait, what am I reading?"

I have this thing about movies. Some might call it an unhealthy obsession. When I was a kid, we didn't go camping or on road trips as a family. We went to Blockbuster instead.

Growing up around movies, I developed preferences. Today I enjoy romantic comedies, thrillers, documentaries about whales, and of course any film involving Tom Hanks, Bruce Willis, or Christopher Walken. *Moulin Rouge* always makes me cry, and I know every line of *Forrest Gump* and Ron Howard's *The Grinch*. I like to picture my life in movie mode because it's way more interesting when James Earl Jones is narrating my every move. I visualize myself as the funny best friend, the quirky sidekick, or even the romantic interest. I don't cast myself as the bad guy. I would love to be the edgy villain, but I would probably apologize for firing a gun or busting down someone's door like a mobster. *Oh my goodness, I am so sorry. Is everyone okay? That was completely uncalled for; let me fix this door frame for you.*

The MRI felt very much like a movie scene, complete with slow-motion shots of plastic hospital curtains swaying behind me as a nurse with a blurry face revealed what we've all waited a third of the book to hear. Maybe it was a Spielberg film, possibly a Tarantino. The scene wouldn't have showed you the six hours that we waited in the stuffy ER room before entering the MRI machine that was shaped like a giant metal donut. It would have cut to the good stuff. It would have cut to the moment shit got real:

*Friday, September 5, 2014, 10:30 p.m.*

INT. SAINT JOSEPH HOSPITAL EMERGENCY ROOM.

SETTING: Saint Joseph Hospital sits amid the urban sprawl of Denver, Colorado, wedged tightly between bookstores and coffee shops, with the towering skyline in the distance. It is late, and the street lights have come on.

MIMI and her MOM sit in a stuffy private room. MIMI is a 22-year-old woman, short in stature, with blue eyes and auburn hair. Her porcelain white skin sometimes tricks people into thinking she is a redhead. But she isn't a redhead. People also ask her if she is allergic to the sun. She dislikes these kinds of questions.

MIMI has been experiencing nausea and dizziness. She is wearing a pale blue gown and sits on the examination table. She is slightly slumped over, as one would be after a long day. MOM sits fidgeting with a pamphlet from the magazine rack in the corner of the room.

A female NURSE enters with a clipboard. MOM puts her pamphlet aside and grips MIMI'S hand tightly.

NURSE:

Ms. Hayes, we're ready for you now.

MIMI rises from the examination table. Camera zooms in on MIMI'S hands detaching from MOM'S slowly.

MIMI:

I'll be fine, Mom.

MOM:

I'll be right here.

MIMI follows NURSE into a dim corridor that leads to a brightly lit room. The room contains a large MRI machine with small tables surrounding it. The machine resembles a giant glazed donut with a skinny table coming out of the hole.

Camera cuts to the table, which is covered in blue medical paper; small tools and cords catch the florescent light. Behind another door is a room separated from the MRI machine room by a glass window. Computer screens are visible inside. NURSE hands MIMI two small orange ear buds.

NURSE:

It gets a little loud in here. You might want these.

MIMI places the ear buds in her ears as NURSE

motions to the examination table. MIMI lies on the table, and NURSE places a large helmet made of plastic over MIMI'S head.

NURSE:

This is so that your head and neck don't move during the procedure. Try your best not to move. Try to relax—take a nap if you can.

Camera fades to NURSE grabbing a needle and IV from the table. Zoom into NURSE taking the cap off the needle.

NURSE:

This is the contrast. It's going to show us what's going on in your brain.

The script would have cut the boring parts, the long minutes spent pondering this question: What *was* going on in my brain? And what exactly they would they contrast? My tendency to over-apologize and my obsessive cleaning habits? My inability to make lasting relationships and my fascination with cheese bread? Perhaps the blue liquid would expose these mysteries too.

NURSE injects MIMI with the needle. MIMI cringes slightly. The blue dye fills the tube, and MIMI watches it enter her arm. NURSE steps into the adjoining room and closes the door.

NURSE (over loudspeaker):

Here we go, Mimi. Once the table moves into the machine, please stay still. Are you ready?

MIMI holds up a hand to make a thumbs-up. The examination table moves slowly into the MRI machine. MIMI'S eyes are wide open. Shadows creep over her face from inside the large metal machine.

Camera cuts to MIMI's view from inside the helmet. She sees buttons and wires and her own breath fogging up the helmet. The machine whizzes and grumbles, and MIMI'S neck muscles tighten. It is dark now. She shuts her eyes tightly.

NURSE:

Mimi? Are you okay? Mimi—

LIGHTS OUT.

Cut to the reveal of the tiny blood berry nestled in my head. I think Spielberg's writer's room would have had fun with this one. The only problem was that this scene was real.

*Your head has exploded and we don't know why, but let me just run out of the room real quick for an undisclosed reason and not return for several hours.*

They'd removed me from the MRI machine and placed me in a small room for the news. I almost wished they'd left me in the machine so that I could scream into the loud container, where no one could hear me. My teeth were chattering.

Goosebumps sprouted all over my body, and I gasped for air like someone had extracted it from the room. The hospital was Alaska. Mom covered me with blankets and more blankets. I had no idea where she was getting all the blankets, but that wasn't important. What was important was the amount of time I had before I became a vegetable. I needed to know when the pain would set in, when my brain would ooze out of my ears and onto the floor. *When does the coma start? Do I get a phone call?*

I couldn't control my shivering body. I was shaking left and right and up and down. There was no rhythm to it. Mom reached for her phone and called Dad. I must have entered a wormhole, because it seemed the minute my mother put down her phone, Dad appeared in the doorway. Time stopped being time. It was simply place; here, in this tiny, cold cube of a room. Here, covered in itchy white blankets with cheesy medical pamphlets all over the walls. It was close to midnight now, and we were still in the room awaiting the return of the nurse. This wasn't in my script. I wasn't supposed to be lying here like a slab of ice, waiting to die.

*Did I just say die?* I was twenty-two. I didn't know what death meant. I didn't know whether I wanted to be cremated or buried. I didn't know what my parents would do with all my shit in the basement. I didn't even know if I believed in heaven or hell. Maybe I would continue to turn into a slab of ice. Maybe I would drift off to sleep. Hopefully wherever I was going had blankets.

I was still contemplating where I could get more blankets, when the nurse appeared. I hadn't actually looked at her before. I'd been looking at the ceiling tiles, the fabric of the blankets, the tissue paper covering the table, anything else. She was tall and slender, and her white coat hung off her like it was on a coat rack.

"You're in stable condition," Coat Rack said. This would have been a great detail to share before leaving the room to do whatever the hell it was she was doing for the past hour and a half.

And I didn't feel stable. I felt unstable, like I could explode at any moment. I wasn't in much pain, though, aside from my usual nausea and dizziness. I was just cold. I could speak, but I saw double when I looked to the left. I wondered if Spielberg would have made the artistic choice to have me howl in pain and fall to the floor, forcing the nurse to pay more attention to me. Tarantino would have had Mom pull out an AK-47 and blow my head off right there to put me out of my misery.

"You can go home now if you want to," she said.

*Coat Rack says what?* She sounded ridiculous. Even if I'd be more comfortable in my own bed, with all my favorite blankets, shouldn't someone be making sure my head didn't explode while I was sleeping? Mom refused to leave until we met with a neurosurgeon, someone who knew how to do a neuro exam and not just put a finger in front of my face and call it a day. The problem was that they wouldn't have a hospital room available until two or three in the morning. Mom and Dad sat back, and we waited some more. I felt like I was at the DMV, holding a number that would never come.

I lay under my pile of sweaty blankets and shut my eyes. My body was tired, but my mind was racing. I tried to organize the tangled information into questions that I wanted answered:

1) What in the actual fuck is going on in our brain right now?

2) Do we have any idea how this happened?

3) Should we be writing down any last words or will or testament or whatever bullshit you're supposed to do when you're eighty-five?

To answer these questions, I had to get inside my own head. I had to know what it looked like in there. I squeezed my eyes shut and pictured a misty garden. Flowers and shrubs and trees wove intricate patterns in the sunlight. A bird sat on a branch and sang to me. I smiled and whistled back to the friendly bird. But as I walked down the path, the garden got dimmer, the mist thicker. Soon the sun was gone entirely, and I was tripping over roots and weeds in the dark. The birds were fleeing the garden en masse; they looked angry now, and black like the stormy sky. Then the weeds latched on to my legs and held me in the middle of the path. I pulled at them and pulled at them, but they wouldn't come loose. More roots attached themselves to my arms and torso, and then a cracking sound came from behind me; I turned to find a wall of water crashing toward me. My legs and arms were still snarled. I couldn't break free. The wall of water roared toward me; the weeds screeched at me like they were alive. The water was dark, almost the color of murky blood. The blood water was approaching me quicker now, just inches from engulfing me—

*Nope. Fuck that garden. I don't like that garden.*

Just as I began picturing my brain as a rocket ship equipped with fancy space suits and moon cheese, Coat Rack came back to inform us that our sixth-floor room was ready. Another nurse who resembled a young Geena Davis carefully sat me and my shaky body in a wheelchair and rolled me into the elevator with Mom and Dad.

The sixth-floor east wing looked like the opening scene to a disease movie, when everyone has evacuated because of the latest deadly monkey germ. It wasn't that the rooms weren't available. The hospital was understaffed. It was a Friday night at two in the morning, and they were ill prepared for my brain bleed. They clearly hadn't cast enough extras for my movie scene. They'd missed their cues.

The neurosurgeon, Dr. Crawford, was not available until Sunday. We sat in my hospital room all weekend waiting to meet him. Mom and Dad took turns sleeping on uncomfortable chairs, resting their wobbly heads on window sills and on each other. I was sure if my parents didn't get answers soon, they'd sue somebody. My ears were throbbing, and my vision had gone all screwy. I kept tripping over my own feet. I was dizzy all the time. I displayed my arm when the nurses told me to and let them stab me with IV needles whenever they wanted. I watched *Back to the Future* on the hospital TV and ate overcooked mac and cheese from the dining hall.

"Good luck finding my veins," I said to the newbie nurse with the needle. "Have you done this before? They're invisible. One nurse ruined a whole bag of IV fluid because she missed the vein." *If you screw this up, I will end you. We have an attorney.*

On Sunday a handsome man in his forties walked into my hospital room as I was attempting to spoon tapioca pudding into my mouth. He had salt and pepper hair and sharp green eyes. His walk was confident and timely. *Spielberg casts well*, I thought. I put my spoon down so as not to embarrass myself.

Dr. Crawford placed a picture up on the wall facing my parents. I craned my neck to see it and closed one eye to compensate for the distorted view. He pointed to a small circular spot in the center of the squishy gray image. "This is your cerebellum," he said. "And this is what we call a cavernous angioma."

*My brain is a cavern! Now I seeeee.* It looked harmless sitting there on the photograph, the tiny clump cavern forming a hole no bigger than a nickel. It wasn't blurry or in motion. It lay on the screen like a lone piece of fruit on a table.

It had hemorrhaged inside my cerebellum on the left side, the doctor said. I didn't even know that my brain could do that kind of thing. I pictured a miniature Grand Canyon filling up with bloody water, and bunnies and lizards running up the walls to escape the flash flood. That did not put me at ease.

Dr. Crawford assured my parents that the bleed was stable and that I should return home to wait for the blood to reabsorb into wherever the hell it came from. After a month we would be able to tell if it had to be fixed.   He was optimistic and calm. He'd seen this injury before and had done similar surgeries in the past.

I looked back to the ceiling tiles, and my eyes glazed over as my parents' heads turned into mumbling clouds. Little IV baggies and pressure cuffs and bunnies trying to run up walls of caverns floated around my consciousness. I lost the ability to believe anything that was said to me. This was another rowboat made of noodles. It wasn't *real*.

## The Dogs Know

The first thing I did after returning home with my new disease was update my Facebook status:

> September 7, 2014, 12:31 p.m.
>
> Update for friends and family: After three long days, many pokes and MRIs, and truly lovely nurse visits, I have been released from the hospital on good behavior. I will be resting at home for the next 3–4 weeks while my brain heals. My stability and vision are still kind of impaired (picture a drunk person, ha-ha), but I am otherwise fine. But don't you think for one second that some silly brain hemorrhage will keep me down. You heard me, Denver Half Marathon; I'm coming for you in October, baby! ☺

I sent it feeling like a champion. Three to four weeks, and I'd leave this disease in the dust like my competition in the half marathon. But… "kind of impaired"? "I am otherwise fine"? I wasn't just a resident of Denialville, I was the fucking mayor.

When I was diagnosed with a cavernous angioma, I was scared out of my gourd. My stumbling off curbs and into student desks wasn't quirky and cute anymore. It was a disease, a living, breathing disease sitting quietly in my brain, waiting to blow. *It had a name now.* And none of this made sense. Dr. Crawford had told me that the clump of cells had formed at birth, creating a vacant space that had caused no harm for my entire life. Until now. Why now? What had I done to myself to earn this new vocabulary?

The thought occurred to me during the diagnosis that the disease was in fact my

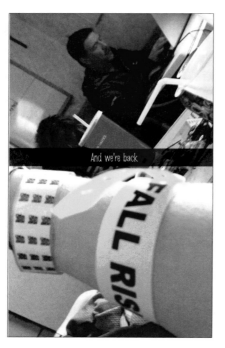

*Friends: "Omg you're in the hospital?"*
*Me: "Didn't you see my Snapchat?"*

doing. That I'd somehow willed my brain to rupture, by sheer determination. It wasn't enough to have a broken spirit. I needed a broken body too. Maybe deep down I wanted this to happen. Maybe I needed to be cut deeper than I already had been by James just months before. But either way, I was humbled in a way that I couldn't describe. I was mortified of my own skin and bones—deceived by them, by everything in the world that I'd come to rely on. Did I voice these fears to my loved ones? Nope. I was too busy laughing, to distract myself from my fear and from the way my body was breaking down before me.

To be fair, when I wrote that Facebook post, it didn't feel like an outright lie. I'd been in a hospital all weekend and was happy to be home and away from IV bags. I had my comfy clothes and my bed and my dog. Now that I'd talked myself out of the initial terror that came with the diagnosis, I could point at my brain injury and laugh. I called it silly and chuckled at how cute and annoying it was in my otherwise fairy-tale life. I became an actor, and Facebook became my platform to play Happy-Go-Lucky Brain-Injured Person.

I'd always been an actor, really. My mother recalls my birth in vivid detail, like all mothers must do to embarrass and lightly shame their kids in front of friends and family. It was Take Your Intern to the Birthing Room Day, and my mother looked up to see twenty clipboards attached to twenty strangers who ogled her as she made a final push to send me out on stage. Since that day I've never, and I mean never, missed a cue.

Surrounded by the likes, comments, and smiley faces, I played this role well now. Almost too well. I faked out my friends and family for months that I was kicking it old school at home with a leaky brain and zero fear of death or destruction. But there was one person I couldn't fool. Okay, so he's not really a person. He's a dog. But he thinks he's a person.

Tucker the Labradoodle saw right through my bullshit Facebook post. The moment I arrived home, he was a changed guy. I was helped out of the car and set gingerly on the couch. He made a perimeter around me, pacing around the living room for several minutes, almost as if calculating the space between each piece of furniture. He came toward me only once and slowly licked the crook of my elbow.

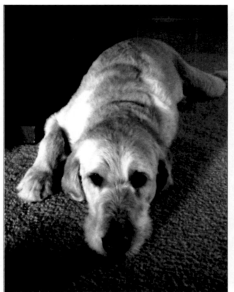 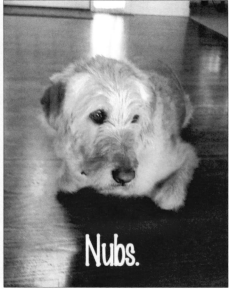

*Sometimes we like to hide our limbs.*

"Hi, buddy!" I smiled.

"What the fuck happened to you?" he might have said back.

I'd never seen Tucker act so strangely. He was gentle and slow. He stopped jumping up on my bed. He stopped opening the door to my room with his nose at odd hours of the night to bother me. When I moved to go down the stairs, he would wait cautiously at the bottom instead of hurtling himself up the steps to shove me over. When I went to bed, he would curl himself in front of the door like he was protecting me from the Brain Boogeyman. He didn't buy into the smiles that covered up my despair. Like Mom, he knew something was not right.

This made me secretly nervous. Where was the line between dogs knowing when you're sick and knowing when you're dying? *Honestly, where is that line?* I needed to know.

Tucker has always been a sensitive guy. He likes the snow but doesn't appreciate the rain; getting him to go to the bathroom on a rainy day is like asking him to gnaw off his own legs. When the Fourth of July comes, he curls up under Mom's armpits and whimpers at every bottle rocket. During loud card games with the family, he turns on his dopey eyes and tries to cuddle with us as we shout and throw cards at one another.

But Tucker has a wild side. He gets too excited about doorbells and tramples people when they come inside the house. He barks at a leaf blowing in the street and stands in front of the refrigerator for hours, waiting for you to get him an ice cube. He does this thing where he gets halfway off my bed and rubs his junk all over my covers as he jumps down. This new and overly sensitive Tucker was not the Tucker I knew. I loved him dearly, but I couldn't source how he knew about my sickness while I was still refusing to come to terms with it. I wondered if he'd sniffed it out in my sleep, me dreaming up a shiny new reality and him connecting the horrifying dots of my future.

Many months later Tucker would visit me in a hospital. Mom brought him in to say hello. When he entered the room, I thought he'd had ass surgery. He looked in worse shape than I did. His legs were squatty and crooked as he limped along, his tail drooping between his legs like a wet rag.

He paraded around the room in misery. This was worse than the Fourth of July. He would sit by Mom for a moment with his paw resting in her hand and sob loudly. I didn't even know a noise like that existed in the animal kingdom. Then he would walk over to the other side of the room, collapse to the floor, and sob some more. Walk to the next corner. Collapse and sob. *Collapseandsobcollapseandsobcollapseandsob.*

I was weirded out by his whimpering in the hospital room. I even laughed at him, pointing at his droopy tail and making fun of his discomfort. It seemed ridiculous that he'd be crying over such a silly thing.

Looking back on it now, I realize that Tucker felt everything—from my sick arrival home from the hospital to my body's quick collapse to my departure to a new hospital and back again. I felt a lot of things too, but I refused to acknowledge them for what they were. I was afraid of becoming a slave to my feelings, afraid of relinquishing my perceived and nonexistent control over my life. I chuckled at any person or animal who admitted their feelings. It was a twisted power play. By not giving way to my emotions, I allowed myself to feel a step above those who did.

I will never know the extent to which Tucker knew. I only know that animals are more intelligent than we give them credit for. Tucker wasn't upset about the wheelchair in the corner of the hospital room because he thought I wouldn't be going on neighborhood walks with him anytime soon. He was upset because he knew deep down that there was a chance I would never be the same again.

Dogs are the best. You throw a ball and they love you for it. You lose sight of love, and they smile that big, goofy smile and you remember all is right with the universe. A dog's love is unmatched by any other love, that I know of, anyway. Tucker would never run off with some other owner—he would never return a love letter unopened. He is the most stable and reliable thing in my life, and I love him more than oxygen. Who else gets excited *every* time I open the door?

Dogs have no way of bullshitting their feelings. They either lick you or they don't.

They either growl at you or they don't. There's no joke to cover up the slobber on your arm.

Tucker was a trooper during my sick days. He was patient, kind, and protective. He knew when to sob in scary hospitals and when to jump on my bed again because I was over the hill to recovery. He showed me the power of unconditional and unrelenting love. Tucker's love could coax me back to life someday, but I had to stop lying to myself first. And to everyone else.

## My Thoughts on Bruce Willis

Bruce Willis has had a very lucrative career. He's one of the only actors I know (I mean, I don't *know* him know him, but I'd like to think if we met we'd agree on a lot of things) who has successfully franchised himself as a friendly neighborhood badass despite natural hair loss. He's been kicking ass and taking names for longer than I've been alive. And Brucey is really good at what he does. He makes dodging flying cars or exploding bombs look like child's play. That is, if your child enjoys assembling weapons of mass destruction and participating in car chases on the freeway, in which case you are nailing this parenting thing.

Sir Willis always takes out his trash. I bet he really does. He has too much respect for the elderly couple across the street to leave those greasy pizza boxes hanging around. He's the kind of guy you wouldn't mind living next door to, even if the Russian mafia does happen to show up every once in a while and crash a stolen vehicle into his living room.

Mr. Willis smokes a lot of cigarettes in his movies, usually while he's bleeding or pointing a gun at someone, sometimes both. Guns don't kill people. Bruce Willis *and* cigarettes kill people. Also, Bruce Willis *with a cigarette in his mouth*. That'll kill you twice.

He's adorable and deadly, and I wish he'd stop being so good at surviving near-death scenarios. This isn't how the world works, just so you know. When I watch Bruce Willis and other crime-fighting actors on the silver screen, I think to myself that there's got to be some injury they're hiding from us. Bruce just leaped off that twelve-story telephone pole and onto a moving car! Just thinking about it snaps my kneecaps in half.

When we ordinary people get in fifty-car pileups, we don't bust out the windshield all fun-like. When we have brain hemorrhages, we don't saunter out of the operating room and still have the energy for a witty retort like "Well *that* went well." No, it did not go well, Bruce. It did not.

As I sat on my couch picking which Netflix series to binge-watch next, I came across *Die Hard*. I'd seen it at least twenty times. But this time as I watched the Big BW wrap his bloody hands in toilet paper and talk nonchalantly to his pal on a walkie-talkie, I realized I wanted to be Bruce Willis *now*. I didn't just want to survive this brain bleed; I wanted to make it my *biiioootch*. If Bruce had been losing blood this entire scene and could still make it through another hour of the movie, then surely I would never break. He was exerting himself; I was sitting on the couch. The blood in my brain would be fine up there.

Bruce is not to blame for these shenanigans. Good ol' Hollywood loves writing the "no flipping way anyone could survive that" scenes. I can't tell you how many times I have believed something would work out fine because I saw it in a movie once. *Leap Year* with Amy Adams convinced me that if I hopped on a flight to Ireland, I would catch myself a witty bartender who was a total babe and would fall head over heels for my quirkiness and inability to remember birthdays. *Julie and Julia*, also with Amy Adams (I think her red hair and light sense of humor are refreshing, so sue me), made me believe that I could cut off all my hair and become a chef. I made a pizza once, and my hair looked awkward once it grew past my shoulders.

This is what acting is all about. It's taking something unbelievable and making it believable. It's the reason I could fool my friends for so long with my brain puns and jokes. The problem is when we buy into Hollywood and make ridiculous choices like racing cars across train tracks, jumping out of airplanes, and even purchasing a fancy glue gun that we know damn well is going to burn us.

But I have always been a cautious person. Even while having pucks shot at my head in ice hockey, I tiptoed around accidents. My only two injuries of note were caused by someone else. So why then did my body collapse doing normal people things like sleeping and watching Netflix? What did Bruce have that I didn't? Was there some *How to Be a Badass and Survive Everything* handbook that I was missing? Where was the YouTube video for this?

I have never claimed to live on any edge. I can't even stand being on the second floor of a hotel. I keep thinking I'm going to tumble down an elevator shaft to my hilarious death. Deep down, I was jealous of Bruce Willis in *Die Hard*. He quite literally made dying hard to do. He laughed off his injuries and made spectacular comebacks. He lost a lot of blood but looked fabulous and rugged by the end credits. I knew that riding a bike without a helmet wasn't a clever idea. I knew that driving 70 in a 40 zone would make me a primetime ass-hat. I knew that turning a corner too quickly with my sensitive brain could land my face on the floor. And I knew that my mother would never approve of any of these unnecessary risks.

But I wanted it. I wanted to be unbreakable, invincible; I wanted to *Die Hard*.

## Gump Walks

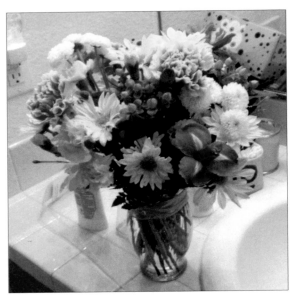

*Very pretty flowers from the cast of 'Til Death Do Us Party*
*that I forgot to water a few times.*

I'd like to say that I spent my initial brain recovery sitting on a park bench, telling everyone that life was like a box of chocolates. In reality, I occupied a bunch of time squatting on see-saws by myself, scaring away the locals. Part of me thought that being the neighborhood cripple was awesome. I could have left the house in fuzzy footie pajamas and a cowgirl hat, and no one would have questioned me. No one.

As part of my post-hospital care, I was required to take three twenty-minute walks a day to maintain blood flow and prevent clotting. With supervision, of course. And a badass walking stick. These mini-walks were supposed to keep my legs strong and my heart pumping blood. In my ignorance, I thought walking would direct the blood away from my brain and into other parts of my body. I'd power walk the problem right out of my head.

What the doctors didn't tell me was that simply walking would not heal the hole in my brain. It was a necessary task, to be sure—remaining sedentary could be damaging—and it didn't hurt that the walking helped distract me. The doctors weren't lying, of course. I just filled in the gaps with my own illogical theories about how quickly my body could heal itself. It was a wait-and-see injury, but my fairy-tale brain had already solved the mystery; I was going to be fine. I had steroids to take and walking to do. In time, the cavernous angioma would stop being a thing.

During my four-week limbo at home, I had constant visits from friends, coworkers, and loved ones. Perhaps my Facebook acting failed, and they sensed something was wrong. But many came under the assumption that I was on the road to recovery, not demise. They brought me chai bread and board games and chick flicks. It was like a vacation to me. I got to see all my friends whenever I wanted. I got unlimited chips and queso.

I imagine this time was harder on everyone else than it was on me. I simply didn't process what was happening to my head or to anything else attached to it. My body began changing faster than I could understand. My left foot developed a drag, and it took me five minutes to open my toothpaste. Every day I grew weaker. Part of me thought this was weird, but I convinced myself that if I just added a few more blocks to my walking route, I could reverse the damage to my atrophying legs.

Sometimes I'd ask my visitors if they wanted to walk me. They'd look at me with raised eyebrows.

"Doctor's orders, man," I'd say. "I have to be walked three times a day. I'm a really needy brain patient."

I felt a little strange about being taken out on walks. I'd never needed to be supervised so closely before. Dr. Crawford explained that it was best due to the dizziness and nausea, the fear being that I'd trip into oncoming traffic and cause more damage, if that was even fucking possible.

Mom started calling my friends Mimi handlers. "All right, you guys," she'd announce to my squad. "She's fragile, so you're going to be her Mimi handlers for today. She likes to go down to the park and back up. But if she gets tired, turn around right away. And take some water in case she gets dehydrated. And here's some sunscreen and a hat. *If you feel a change in pressure, a mask will fall from the sky and inflate with air...*"

Tucker was not enthused by the Mimi handler situation. Every time I'd get my shoes and my handler ready to go, he'd pace the room or try to hide my cane. I thought it was because I was robbing him of his walks, and he couldn't come to terms with it. As we all know, he was up to his floppy ears with worry.

With my walking stick that Dad found for me at a thrift store and my parade of Mimi handlers, I felt like Forrest Gump in his running days. I'd had my days in 'Nam and I loved Jen-nay a lot, but now it was time to move. Anytime I got tired after a block or two, I would stop and turn to whichever friend I was with.

"I think I'm done walking now," I'd say in true Gump fashion, and pivot back for home.

I'd order my handler to help me reenact this scene; I had it down to an exact science. I'd have them pretend to be completely put out, like I had just walked them across the countryside and suddenly decided to turn around. Many of my friends obliged. A few thought I was insane.

~

As my condition worsened, walking around the block became more difficult, and I stumbled on rocks and off sidewalks. My vision was getting worse. I had to focus really hard on each movement so that I could see where I was going.

"If anyone was looking for the curb," I would say, "I found it." My friends laughed uncomfortably with me and watched in terror as I became less and less like myself.

Erin and my mother were my evening shift Mimi handlers. These walks involved more life contemplation than joking; it was here that I noticed my very unfunny loss of freedom and began to get outwardly emotional. My feet wouldn't do what my brain told them to do. I was relying more heavily on the cane. This situation was getting less funny with each wonky step on the pavement, and my temper ran high.

Early one evening during week three of the post-diagnosis Gump walking parade, I went out with Erin for my third walk of the day. The sun was just setting. I was tired and didn't want to go, but I wanted my brain bleed to go away, so I shoved my shoes onto my feet and grabbed my cane. It had been several weeks since my diagnosis, and things weren't looking any better. I couldn't see an end in sight.

"How do you feel?" Erin asked as we puttered around the corner.

"I feel like shit," I said. "Absolute shit."

"It could always be worse."

"I'm sorry, what?"

"I said it could be—"

"I fucking heard what you said." I gripped my cane tighter. "But how exactly could this be worse, Erin?" James was gone, and it still stung. My head was bleeding, and it wasn't improving. I knew that people were dying of cancer and AIDS. I knew that people had worse breakups or had lost loved ones to car accidents. But what the fuck was she talking about?

I started to cry. "You don't know how I feel or what I'm going through," I said. "You will never know any of this. You can't say things like that to me! I can't fucking walk, and James left me for somebody else!" I was screaming in her face now. I took my walking cane and chucked it at her and stormed off in the opposite direction. I threw my functioning middle finger at her as I waddled down the street.

I didn't get very far before I needed my cane back. Erin joined me after giving me a few minutes to cool down, and apologized, and we walked the next two blocks in silence. Her words confused me. I didn't know how I felt about sympathy or empathy or denial or humility. I was still finding ways to joke on Gump walks, but other times these walks made me angry. My body wasn't working the way it was supposed to. I couldn't train for my half marathon, and I wasn't teaching. I was just the neighborhood cripple.

I see now that Erin was trying to comfort me in her own way. She shared my pain on some level and wanted to make it better. After all, she'd been volunteering as a Mimi handler for weeks. She was putting in time and making an effort to console me. She was doing the best that she could.

After my walk with Erin and the middle finger, I interpreted her words in a new way. Maybe it wasn't such a big deal now that I couldn't walk gracefully around the block. What if in a few months I lost the ability entirely? What if I went numb from the neck down? What if I had to be fed through a straw? Who would love me then? Would I ever have the chance to meet my Prince Charming for real?

I had a lot of questions about my future. I harbored plenty of uncertainty and fear. I had to give myself permission to feel these things, and I wasn't willing to do that. I also didn't think it would make anyone happy if I let myself talk that way, and I certainly wasn't ready to let the emotional tsunami hit me, because then I'd actually have to deal with this shit. And while Erin's words hurt because I felt that she wasn't being sensitive to my world, they made me think myself into an even darker hole.

I wasn't Bruce Willis. I wasn't invincible at all. Maybe things really could get worse.

And maybe they would.

## Late-Night Fries and MRIs with Dad

"I can't feel on the left side of my tongue," I said abruptly during a Gump Walk with Erin one evening. "That's normal, right?" I was laughing at myself. Erin was not.

"What?" Apparently she needed clarification of whatever fucked-up shit just came out of my laughter.

I pointed to my tongue. "Just on the left side. I can't taste anything over there."

"How long has this been going on?" she asked.

"Like a week," I said. "It's fine. It's normal."

The first time I'd noticed a lack of taste, I was sipping ginger ale through a straw. It felt strange, like the bubbly fizz was gone. I ignored it for a while. I wasn't eating a whole lot anyway. But the morning of that Gump Walk, I'd attempted Captain Crunch, and I was pretty sure I should have been able to taste the sugary sweetness on my tongue. Later I'd experimented with a few more spoonfuls and discovered that just the left side was numb. I could talk fine other than a tiny slur with a few words, and my face wasn't drooping. I could still wear my mask of lies.

At this point in the conversation, Erin turned around and walked me the block and a half home, looking peeved. *Why is she so upset? This is supposed to be hilarious.* Erin demanded that I tell our parents about the new symptom immediately. I rolled my eyes. I didn't want to make a big deal out of it; I just wanted Erin to be in on the joke. It hadn't occurred to me yet that this funny numb tongue business could be for good. That I might not ever be able to taste again. But I laughed at this too. I put Bruce Willis up on my shoulder like a badass guardian angel and turned to him for witty comebacks: *At least you still have the right side, kid.*

I'd read up on brain damage, of course. I'd googled *cavernous angioma* from the confines of my bed many times before. I knew damn well that the odds were against me. All these new and very unfunny symptoms could be permanent. Would I be able to laugh if my entire mouth went numb? Could I still make jokes? Would life even be worth living if I couldn't taste extra-sharp cheddar?

When we got back to the house, I told Mom and Dad about my tongue. Mom had Dr. Crawford's office on speed dial and handed me the phone to talk to a nurse because he was in a meeting. I left a message with her that the left side of my tongue was numb and that I guess I thought that was a little weird. She scheduled a second MRI for later in the week and said they would call back to ask more questions about my taste buds.

The days before the next MRI passed by in an uneasy rhythm. I had plenty of Netflix to watch, abundant movies to displace me from my spiraling reality. But no matter how many quirky rom-coms I watched, I couldn't shake the fact that I'd now lost two senses. By this point I saw double regularly, and that made me dizzy and unstable the few times I was in motion. Now I couldn't taste on half of my tongue. I negotiated which of my senses could go next, which one I liked the least of the five: hearing, sight, touch, smell, taste. Brucey would have told me how *two outta five ain't bad*, but it was bad. Really bad. It was scary enough to have one of these impaired. Now I was trying to determine which one I'd rather sell in a garage sale.

The MRI was scheduled for nine thirty at night in a location we'd never heard of about forty minutes from our house. The place didn't even look open.

"Are you sure this is right, Dad?" I asked as we parked in an abandoned lot.

"Looks like it." He held me up by my right arm as we shuffled to the double doors. He'd recently injured his right knee playing hockey. When the two of us walked arm in arm, we looked like wobbly little non-ambi-turners. We quoted *Zoolander* and made jokes daily that neither of us could turn left. He was humoring me. He was hurting too.

When we got inside, Dad grabbed me a wheelchair he found in a corner. I didn't want to need it, but I did. The cane was becoming its own obstacle now that my hands struggled to hang on to it, let alone use it properly. Dad popped a few wheelies on the way to the radiology department to make me feel better about being put in another big metal tube. We saw no one in the halls or at any of the desks. I wondered what kind of people worked these shifts at hospitals, what kind of madman would be interpreting my brain scans at this hour.

We were met by a rather alert woman with a clipboard. I'd started to hate clipboards, those stupid brown things that clamped together bad news with more bad news. I made a mental note to steal one and smash the living daylights out of it sometime behind a plastic curtain.

"Checking in?" she said.

I reached for my health insurance card and driver's license, but there was a holdup. The fingers on my left hand were taking their sweet time following my brain's orders to pull the slippery things out of my wallet. I tried using my right hand, my dominant hand, to help the other. But that one was slow too. I floundered for several seconds with the task of taking them out and then struggled to push them across the counter. These increasingly apparent symptoms put me on edge. Already this MRI visit felt much different from the first. There were no fairy tales, no movie scenes, no overprotective motherly instincts here. I was checking in. I had an appointment. They were looking for something bigger now, something strange.

~

I know a lot about medical imaging. I know about X-rays because one time some neighborhood kids double-jumped me off the trampoline and I broke my arm. Freaking punks. I know about CAT scans too. When I was two years old, I walked behind Erin as she was swinging a metal baseball bat in our grandparents' backyard. That fractured my cheekbone and got me a cool black eye that made my parents look like awful people in the grocery store. I had to sit in a big machine and be completely still so that they could take pictures of my tiny broken cheeks. I'm also pretty sure those fancy X-ray machines at the airport can read your mind, but that's a separate conversation we should have behind closed doors.

We've come a long way in the medical field. It's only recently that technology has advanced enough to show what's going on deep inside our gooey bodies. Up until now, brain surgeries were a high-stakes game of Operation. The board game from the '90s, that is. It wasn't uncommon for a surgeon to drill a hole in your head without understanding what would happen next. Medical imaging is amazing. It saves lives, and it most certainly saved mine.

But just because we can see what's in there, doesn't mean we'll understand. After finally being taken seriously enough to get the first MRI, I'd had hopes that they would find something conclusive. Perhaps they'd uncover the secrets to the universe in there. Or they'd find the faulty wire that had been causing all my dysfunctional relationships. If nothing else, they'd figure out what in the hell they needed to do about that little blood bubble. Instead, it was maybes. *Maybe* this blood will go back to normal. *Maybe* it will not go back to normal. *Maybe* you'll realize that you're not Bruce Willis and stop trying to hop over your couch like it's a moving car.

I wasn't sure what they were looking for this time. A lot had changed in a few weeks. I'd lost a majority of mobility on the left side of my body and started slurring words in the past few days too. But a lot had also stayed the same. A part of me still thought I needed James. Or maybe not James, but the idea of James. I was surrounded by friends and family, yet still I was lonely. I was given gifts and chocolates and balloons, but I remained empty. All my parents' love, my friends' gifts and affection––none of that could mend the massive hole I'd ripped inside myself. This hole had nothing to do with my cavernous angioma or the havoc it was causing in my body. And though neither could be cured with an imaginative story or a fictional movie character, this hole could not be seen with a fancy metal tube or subdued with bed rest and walks around the block. This was a different part of my brain entirely—an area that needed its own form of surgery. There was something in there, all right. And I needed them to find it.

~

After finally unearthing my documents from my wallet, I was taken down to the metal tube. Dad gave me one last thumbs-up as they wheeled me out of the waiting room: "I'll be right here." I had no doubts. He always was, and Mom too. They were always there.

The nurse wheeled me away through a set of double doors. It wasn't a movie scene here either—it was too familiar. And it was too quick. The first MRI had taken forty-five minutes; this one took fifteen. If it were in a movie, it would have been a quick blip on the screen, no dramatic music, no character development. Before I could process which sounds I was listening to, they pulled me out. They removed the large plastic helmet from my head and told me they'd call me soon. I felt like I was on an awkward date. *Sorry, family emergency. No, I'll call you. Could you grab the check?*

I was wheeled back into the waiting room, where I found Dad fiddling with a magazine.

"That was quick," he said. "Everything go okay?"

"Just your standard metal tube," I said. "I'm hungry."

"What do you want?"

"French fries."

Boy, did I want French fries. I'd never wanted anything so bad in my life. I hadn't had an appetite in weeks, so I had to capitalize. My dad knew this too.

It was close to ten o'clock by the time we got to the car, and most of our go-to French fry eateries were already closed. But Dad soldiered on. We drove around for another ten minutes before we finally spotted the golden arches of a McDonalds. I was ecstatic.

"Hello, welcome to McDonalds, what can I get for you tonight?" the tiny box said.

"Two large fries and a—what do you want to drink?"

"Sprite," I said, and rested my head outside the window. "I'm dizzy."

"A large Sprite, please," Dad said.

I kicked back my seat to relax. I was happy to be hungry, but I was exhausted and dizzy still. I needed those fries to get in my belly and stay there. But I needed more than the salt and trans fats tonight. I needed to find myself again.

## What Doesn't Kill You Makes You Skinnier, Part Two

The thigh gap is a unicorn. It is not a thing. Victoria's Secret would have you believe that the average woman's thighs do not touch. But they do. I can show you every pair of jeans I own; the thighs are destroyed, because my thighs are meant to touch each other. All my pants look as though someone took a cheese grater to my crotch. And this is okay.

It came as quite a shock when I acquired this stupidly sought-after gap after the onset of my brain symptoms. As a hockey player of eight years and an active runner, I'd always been proud of my gam-gams, however tiny and nubbly they were compared with literally anyone else's. But these were not the legs of an athlete. They were the legs of a sick person. I'd been training for a half marathon, and now I had Tiny Tim legs. Minus the miniature leg braces. And maybe soon enough I'd need those too.

In addition to the thigh gap, I gained a fat face. Don't even try to deny it, friends who are reading this who tried to lie to me about the balloon face. I was very disproportional. I mean, I always have been. But now I looked like a garden gnome who'd gotten shrink-wrapped everywhere but the face.

The weight and muscle mass that exited my legs made a curious appearance in my face due to the steroids I was taking to deflate the swelling in my brain. I'd hardly bothered reading the labels on the medicine bottles, but I doubted they read "Your face may get the size of a double-decker bus. Please take with plenty of water." Amid my attempts to make fun of terrifying things, I wrote a haiku about it. *Ahem:*

My face it is fat
My cheeks are like round balloons
My face it is fat

Writing the poem kept my brain preoccupied, but underneath the guise was unprocessed fear. My body was changing quickly again, quicker than I could comprehend, and deep down I knew that it was disturbing. I'd gotten scary-skinny at summer camp. But this time it was unwanted. I wasn't trying to compete with Molly the Trollop. I wasn't trying to be the most brain-damaged-looking person on the block. I didn't want the chicken legs or the fat face. I wanted to not be sick anymore.

At home I wore a lot of sweatpants. I didn't bother putting a bra on if none of my friends were coming over that day. I might go a few days without showering. It seemed cumbersome and unnecessary; the hot water made me dizzy, and my mother got stressed every time I showered upstairs without telling anyone. Eventually she told me to start showering downstairs next to Dad's office so that he could be there if I slipped and fell.

For a while my friends would stop by to get me out of the house. Like a field trip. I couldn't drive anymore. I couldn't go to the movies because it hurt my eyes too much and crowds made me anxious. My field trips had expiration dates. *Try to find a quiet corner of the restaurant and leave if it gets loud. She can't do loud.* Mom was always very clear on directions for how to handle little frail me.

Unlike with my heartbreak, I couldn't manage this depression with running ten miles and drinking a gallon of coffee. I couldn't do anything. The one muscle I was using was my right thumb to change the channel on the TV. My heart was sinking faster into the couch than I was. I couldn't exercise to get endorphins. I couldn't go on dates, nor did I want to. The outside world seemed alien and loud to me now. It wasn't safe out there. But the atrophy wasn't safe either.

I'd had the opportunity to smother myself in self-love. I could have given myself time to heal the right way, to care for myself and give my body what it needed. Several months ago I'd had the chance to dedicate my life to the things that made me feel alive. Instead, I'd dated too many strangers and starved myself of nourishment. I'd run away from my problems and myself. *You're not good enough for James. You're not good enough for you.*

Now I was overwhelmingly incapable of loving myself in this state. I walked around the block less and less and watched enough Netflix to entertain a small village for a year. Every so often a friend would come by and see me at my newest low. They'd hide their shock and try to cheer me up. They'd take me on field trips to get sushi and buy blouses that I wouldn't wear.

But none of this could soothe my growing desire to change who I was becoming. In a few days, I would hear back from Dr. Crawford's office about my last MRI. I needed this news, good, bad, or ugly. I needed it more than I'd needed anything before.

## Pulling a Presley

When asked how we want to kick the bucket, we all answer with something poetic like "at the top of a mountain with a handful of flowers to throw in the wind at sunset" or "in the arms of Patrick Dempsey." If all doctors looked like McDreamy, I wouldn't have anxiety about hospitals. I'd probably throw myself down a set of stairs daily if I knew there'd be a hottie putting in my IV or changing the bandages on my new head wound. Everyone wants to die in a beautiful way. No one wants to die on a toilet.

A few days after my MRI and French fry session with Dad, the highly anticipated phone call came from Dr. Crawford's office. I was instructed to come in to meet with Dr. C to discuss the results in person. This didn't sound good. Mom and Dad drove me over that day, and we sat in a little dark room to look at the before and after shots of my beautifully broken brain.

"This was the first MRI we took when we diagnosed you," the doctor said, pointing to a squishy image on the right. "And *this* is the MRI we took the other day." He pointed to the left.

Both images had a circular spot to the left of my cerebellum. This was the hemorrhage, a pooling of blood inside a clump of cells, caught on camera by some lab technicians during the late shift. However, the image to the left's circle was bigger, this time getting closer to what Dr. C called the brain stem. For those who don't know, the brain stem controls that thing we do all the time that keeps us alive. You know, *breathing*. This was kind of a big deal. A "we hope you don't die any minute now" big deal.

"We'd like you to come in for surgery," Dr. Crawford said. "On Friday."

I thought about my little whiteboard calendar in my bedroom. On Friday I was probably going to continue binge-watching *How I Met Your Mother*. I was most likely going to try typing more funny commentary on my brain damage. I'd definitely eat a bunch of junk food that I couldn't taste. *Yeah, I guess I could squeeze in a quick brain surgery on Friday. I suppose I'll pencil that in…for…*

Three days from now. It was Tuesday.

Dr. Crawford had done this before, which made one of us. He told my parents and me where he'd "make an incision" and how he'd "extract the blood" from the hole in my skull. It sounded ridiculous. Like he'd be dumping holy water on my head and performing an exorcism. His delivery of the words was calm and calculated. He explained the risks of the procedure and possible worst-case scenarios, like an induced coma or several more weeks of recovery. My parents were soothed by this speech. I fixed my gaze on the glossy photographs.

I was confused by my jumbled-up feelings. So much had happened between Brain 1 and Brain 2. I'd added more symptoms to my fancy hospital rap sheet, and I'd watched a hell of a lot of Netflix that I couldn't see properly. I was troubled by this side-by-side narrative thrust before my half-working eyes. And there was so much more to come.

Dr. Crawford handed me a pamphlet about my upcoming appointment as we exited the doctor's office. I tried to scan it with my right eye for meaning.

"Do you mind if we stop at East really quick?" I asked my parents, shoving the pamphlet in my bag as we walked slowly to the car. If I was going to have my brain exorcism on Friday, now would be an appropriate time to inform them.

"Sure, sweetheart," Mom said gently.

The high school was only a block from Dr. Crawford's office. I didn't know why I wanted to go visit Lindsay and my students so badly—I looked like a beaten-down zombie from *The Walking Dead.* Maybe I needed to say it out loud for it to really be true. I didn't realize until much later that I was putting on the funny mask one more time to reassure myself that I'd be okay.

I hobbled up the grand staircase and knocked at room 238. Cody opened the door.

"Ms. H?" he said, mouth gaping.

"Hi, you guys! Just stopping in to say hello!"

Lindsay looked horrified. She airlifted me a chair, and I took several minutes to sit in it properly.

"What's that?" Kylie said, pointing to the stick in my feeble hands.

"This is my walking cane!" I said. "Isn't it cool, you guys?"

I could count on one skinny hand how many interactions I'd had with these kids. The idea that I could show up now and announce my brain surgery like some kind of fucked-up accomplishment was insane. There was no reason to be here other than my delusion that I'd be back in the classroom on Monday with a cool scar and a story. But the kids took the news well and asked questions. Their curious eyes examined my fragile body. One brave soul asked what we were all thinking: "Are you going to *die*, Ms. H?"

"Oh no, sweethearts!" I smiled like a giant liar. "No way. I'm going to be just fine."

I'd not only lied to my students, I'd lied to myself. I was *fine*? Why did I feel the need to scare the living shit out of them like that? I didn't want their sympathy, just like I didn't want to miss an episode of *How I Met Your Mother* for this stupid brain surgery. Maybe I'd just wanted the laughs. The uncomfortable "wait, are you about to die right now?" laughs.

About eight o'clock that night, I went to the bathroom to sit on the toilet and think about my life choices. And also to take a poop, as one does.

I have had a variety of fainting spells in my life, ranging from passing out at local blood banks to falling into a trash can while watching a nurse change out my grandmother's IV. I've always turned green at the thought of bodily fluids, and my dad is convinced that I'll never be able to have children if I don't snap out of it. It's not that I mean to be this way; my body just tells itself that we're dying and falls to the floor.

As I sat on the pot, I felt sick to my stomach, more so than usual for this type of activity. I was lightheaded too. My heartbeat sped up, and then all sounds became muffled. Next would be dark spots surrounding the room, and then unconsciousness, I was sure of it. I'd been passing out in doctor's offices and during health class videos since before I could remember. This wasn't my first time at the rodeo. I knew the routine and could usually avoid smacking my head on the floor if I reacted soon enough.

The only problem was that I was shitting. I was shitting on the toilet and was about to pass out. This was not the normal setting for this kind of thing. More terrifying than the toilet was the quickly surfacing idea that these could be my last moments on earth. My brain was already bleeding, so how far a stretch could it be that my hemorrhage had hit my brain stem? Dr. C had mentioned this earlier, but now it kicked in. Within seconds I'd considered the possibility that tomorrow would not arrive. Pretty deep for a Tuesday night shit.

I'd never truly contemplated my mortality before. I'd been joking about it nonstop since my diagnosis, but this time was different. I had a google-able disease. This time I really could be dying. On a toilet. My last moments could be spent going poop. I was embarrassed. And I was really, really scared. I'd just found out I'd be having brain surgery on Friday. What if my brain and I didn't have a second date? Was I going to die then? Or what if I died now, three days from the finish line and shitting on this toilet?

Time slowed down. I thought about Elvis. He'd died on a toilet. The King had died taking a shit. Extraordinary people often died in ordinary ways, but death seemed so much scarier when it came for you in the mundane, the commonplace and everyday. And who's to say my body would stop pooping once I died? I'd be written into the history books as just another toilet dead person. A dirty, dirty death. Bruce would be really disappointed.

I breathed in heavily, the dark surrounding me now. Time was speeding up again. I didn't have time to think about how embarrassing this was or whether I'd have seven seconds of postmortem thought. I could hear my own heart pounding. Elvis wigs and white, bejeweled bell-bottoms flooded into my brain as distant objects just out of reach. *I'm going to have unfinished business*, I thought. *Literally*. I went from trying to negotiate humor to utterly terrified in seconds.

*BANG.*

The next thing I remember was Erin's voice asking me if I was okay. She must have heard me hit the floor and come over to check on me. My nose was touching the door. I didn't know how long I'd been there or if any bodily fluids were still coming out.

"Don't—don't come in here, okay?" I said. "Go get Mom!" I peered around my body to see if I had made a mess of the floor. Seemed like I'd held it in just in time for my body to collapse off the toilet and onto the cold tile. I didn't know who to thank—god, Buddha, my own body. But whoever was in charge, I was grateful and shaken.

I cleaned myself up and regained my composure. Mom knocked on the bathroom door and came in looking horrified. I told her that I'd passed out but didn't think I'd hit my head. Then I crawled into bed, feeling like the luckiest person alive to have survived a deadly encounter with my toilet. Mom tucked the covers around me.

"If you need anything, let me know," she said. "I'm right here."

I had to chuckle so that I wouldn't burst into tears all over my pillow. Would she always be there? Would I? I slipped into a quasi-slumber. My brain surgery was just days away: Friday, October 3, 2014. I wasn't sure yet if the date would be etched on a gravestone or timestamped in an obituary. But whatever happened, this date would change me forever.

## Last Supper Beef Fest

*Thursday, October 2, 2014, 6:02 a.m.*

I was awake. And I was hungry. With my right eye I glanced at the tiny orange bottle of medication on my bedside table. The past few days, my double vision had ramped up, so I'd gotten into the habit of closing the other eye so that I could see monocular. It was worse in the mornings.

The medicine bottle didn't look appetizing. But then again, nothing did these days. I rolled over. I didn't want to look at the bottle anymore. *My brain medicine.* I didn't care that it could be keeping me alive. I wasn't even positive what it was doing in there that was so important. But I knew one thing: It was keeping me awake. And it was making me hungry, which was strange, considering I didn't want to eat anything.

My body certainly needed nourishment. I looked like a skeletal runway model, minus the intense eyebrows and graceful runway walk. But I was hungrier than that. I needed more than food. I wanted to be done with the medicine bottles and doctor's visits and MRIs. I craved attention that wasn't cloaked in sympathy from strangers and loved ones. This wasn't a romantic "I'll stay with you even if you're dying" movie. I didn't want a first date montage; I wanted to make it to the end credits with someone who loved because I was alive, not because I was dying.

Gifts and well-wishes came in a steady flow in the days leading up to my brain's big moment. Mom forced me to write down who gave me what so that I could send thank you letters afterward. This was encouraging. She'd committed herself to the idea that the surgery would go well, which meant thanking Grandma for the get-well cookies was imperative. I wasn't as sure, but I still had twenty-four hours to stew over it as I sorted through my gifts and baked goods.

Around noon that day, a gigantic box of frozen meats arrived at my doorstep. It sounds like I'm making this up. But it was a thing, you guys, a real thing. The doorbell rang, and Tucker attacked the front door like his life depended on it. A delivery guy handed over a box to Erin and she signed for me.

"Don't get up," she said.

"Wasn't planning on it," I called from the couch. "What is it?"

"Maybe it's worse than we thought," she said, examining the box. "I guess you're getting a last supper tonight, Memes."

She brought the box over to me with a pair of scissors. The box read "Omaha Steaks" in big red letters.

"What is this?" I asked.

"Let's open it and find out."

We cut open the box to find frozen burgers, gourmet franks, baked potatoes, and filet mignon…hold it right there. *Filet mignon.* If anyone ever sends filet mignon to your doorstep, you marry them.

"Dad?" I called to his office door.

"Who sent me a box of meats?"

"What?" He came into the kitchen.

"Look, someone sent me a *box of meats.*" I shook a frozen bratwurst at him.

He read the name on the side of the box. "Those are my contractors and civil engineers."

Sadly I could not marry my father's contractors and civil engineers, because they had wives and kids, but I wanted to. Surely they'd have understood that this was the closest thing to a marriage proposal I'd ever had and were prepared to put an onion ring on it.

On the inside of the box was a personalized note: "We hope this grilled goodness brightens your day!"

I looked at it in awe. Friends of my dad had sent me all I could ever ask for: *a box of meats to grill*. I didn't care that I couldn't grill. Or even walk. I opened the box of meaty glory and analyzed its contents: fancy meats, expensive meats, meats wrapped in other meats. If I ever had to have a last supper, this would surpass all expectations.

But I couldn't eat the meats that day. Dad told me no.

"Why not?" I asked in shock, holding the plastic-wrapped meats in my arms like a tiny child.

"Let's save it," he said. "For when you get home, when you're better."

I was disappointed that I wouldn't be eating grilled meats the night before my brain surgery. It felt like a reasonable last request. If something went wrong in that surgery room, I wanted to know I'd had filet mignon one last time. But Dad's words were also reassuring. He denied me the box of meats because he refused to believe it really would be my last supper. Just like Mom made me write thank you cards.

"They'll be here when you get back," he said. From where, I didn't know.

I slouched back on the couch in defeat.

The rest of the day, I was antsy. I couldn't eat my meats, and I had to answer phone calls all day from friends and family who were "wishing me a good surgery." The problem was that I didn't want to "have a good surgery," like something monogrammed into a muffin tin. I didn't want to think about this stupid surgery at all.

"Yep, Grandma, it's going to go great. I'm not worried—"

"Sure, Cousin, I'll text you when I'm done. Yeah, thanks for the fruit basket—"

"Dude, I got a box of meats in the mail today—"

The hours ticked away, and I wasn't out climbing a mountain or writing something profound in my diary. I was answering phone calls from worried people and talking them down off the panicked surgery ledge. I was puttering around the house, bored and wishing I could have my meats. This wasn't the kind of possibly last day I'd seen portrayed in the movies. Those people all did something meaningful and grand. I was just a loser with a box of meats I couldn't grill.

I didn't want this surgery. It was like the medicine bottle on my bedside table. I hated it, but I knew I needed it. I was supposed to be excited, or so my parents had implied. While they harbored their own fears, they were relieved to be taking action. The sitting and waiting had atrophied them too.

The hours sped up and slowed down. When I wanted the surgery to hurry up and get there, time was slow. When I wanted it to not happen so I could enjoy the day, the hands on the clock spun so fast, they popped off the wall.

At six o'clock the doorbell rang, snapping me back to my remaining senses. But this time it wasn't a box of grilled meats. It was something—or rather, some*one*--else.

# #YOLO

People throw around hashtags like birthday confetti. They can be a lot of fun and make even the simplest of occasions feel like a trip to the grocery store on LSD. But they can also be annoying as fuck and make a total mess of your social media pages and/or living room.

One of my least favorite hashtags is #YOLO. This means "You only live once." People under the age of thirty use it when they think they are living on the edge, or when they are being stupid under the disguise of spontaneity. Dads use it to feel hip. And while I like to believe that I will be reincarnated as a sultan or a sheik or a white male with privilege, I don't have a lot of science to prove that we'll be coming back for a reprise once we die. Sorry, still working on it.

This hashtag stirred up something within me in the days leading up to my surgery. I knew deep down that #YOLO was true. I was young enough to want immortality but smart enough to know that I needed to wear my seatbelt. But for years people had been using #YOLO to explain the most moronic and irresponsible of behaviors, some of which I'd partaken of myself: texting and driving, binge-drinking, and the like. It was as if nobody really knew that you *actually* only lived once. Especially not me.

The evening before my surgery the doorbell rang, and it wasn't a box of meats or a card or a bouquet made of pineapples. It was my good friend Maurice. Maurice, "Moe," and I had met through James several years before—before James and I parted ways, before I lost motor functions and my sense of self. Moe was at ground zero when I got sick; he was there from the beginning of it all, back when my symptoms were still explained to me as depression and paranoia.

Moe: Hey girlie, how you doin'?

Mimi: Not entirely sure. I just passed out in my doctor's office…
that's normal, right?

Moe: Um no. What's going on?

Mimi: They don't know. Idiots. I'm picking up some drugs.

Mimi:…by drugs I mean Dramamine. Borrrrriiiiing.

Moe was a birthmark. He was there for every Gump Walk and ice cream binge, and he never asked anything of me during these visits, other than which romantic comedy I wanted to watch as my parents ordered pizza for us. I usually wore my stained pajamas and couldn't remember the last time I'd washed my hair. He'd say I looked great. I probably didn't.

Tonight when Moe rang the doorbell, my parents greeted him like he was the president. They smiled brightly, apologized for the nonexistent mess, and got him a Pepsi from the fridge within seconds of him entering the house. He is a hero to them, and I suspect my mother really wants us to get together, even though he's about ten years older than I am.

Mom and Dad made sure that Moe was comfortable as I puttered around the kitchen with my cane, thinking about what to eat for dinner. I still wasn't allowed to have the meats, which I made very vocal to Moe as I knocked things around the pantry loudly. Anything but the filet mignon sounded disgusting, but I knew I had to eat now because my surgery required a twelve-hour fast beforehand. It would be a long twelve-plus hours without my filet mignon.

I decided on a frozen burrito just as the doorbell rang again. This time it was Brittney, another friend I'd met from James's time working at the airport and a close friend of Moe's. Moe jumped up to herd her into the house as my parents grabbed more beverages.

"No caffeine for you," Mom said to me and handed a Pepsi to Brit. "Big day tomorrow."

The microwave beeped, and I moved slowly from the table.

"I'll get it!" Brit said.

"No, really, I'll be there in a minute." I shuffled in embarrassment. If we weren't doing a steak cookout, then I sure as shit wanted to make my own frozen burrito.

The doorbell rang again and again, each time announcing a new person from a different era of my life. There was Hayley from elementary school, Riley and Shannon from high school, and Ana, Brit, and Moe from the airport crew. It's entirely possible I'm forgetting a few people in this kitchen scene. If you've been excluded, please accept my sincerest apologies for my lack of memory. I probably should have kept track of my visitors along with my gift baskets. Your thank you card is in the mail.

My entire kitchen was filled with my past. Many of the people sitting around the table with me didn't know each other. They made introductions as Mom and Dad flitted about the room, making sure everyone had a beverage with the right amount of ice. I sat eating my soggy burrito and struggling to use my fork correctly. And trying not to think about the kind of knives they'd be using to open my skull.

It didn't occur to me in that moment, but death was all around me. It was right next to me at the dinner table. Every one of my friends had had near-death misses: in cars or crossing the street with headphones on. Once my little brother almost choked to death on a piece of cheese, and my dad had to do a mini-Heimlich maneuver. Large-scale or seemingly insignificant—it didn't matter. We'd all survived a close brush with death. My family and friends were survivors.

When we survive these near disasters, we exhale deeper than we ever have and thank our lucky stars that we're alive. It's terrifying to think we could have been done for if we'd been a mere inch to the left or the right—to recognize that we are tiny cogs in a giant machine moving at top speed in an unpredictable world. But these deep contemplations seldom last very long. We don't run out of our office cubicles all Jimmy Stewart-like, exclaiming, "Look, everyone! I am alive and breathing in this beautiful world! Isn't that great?!" But we really should.

The night before my brain surgery, I was still making fun of my situation, pretending I was not going to have invasive and unpredictable surgery the next day. If I repeated the information for long enough, I could add it to my comedy routine. *On a scale of one to Ryan Gosling, how sexy is my surgeon, amirite? Do you think I get to keep my underpants on during surgery?*

"Are you nervous for tomorrow?" Brit asked.

"Nervous?" I said. "Nah, man. They're just going in there with an ice cream scoop." My audience looked at me with awkward smiles, the kind that usually accompany what we in the comedy business call bombing.

But then my stomach dropped like a WMD. As I sat at the dinner table, eating my microwaved burrito sloppily and cracking jokes to my pals, weird thoughts filtered through my brain. *Are all these friends coming out to see me because I'm not going to survive this surgery tomorrow? Oh…shit.* Of course I had heard the neurosurgeon mention this possibility several days before, along with other frightening outcomes, including waking up with a straw coming out of my head. But I hadn't actually thought about this, or at least had come to terms with what it meant. As far as I had concerned myself, the straw situation would be hilarious.

I shifted back in my chair, and my head slumped to the side. Once my audience left, it would be just me and the burrito and my bleeding brain. I put my fork down and observed my friends separately. It was time. I stood up slowly, and one by one they hugged me and wished me well. Hayley gave me a bag filled with blankets and candy. Parting gifts and goodbyes for the Hopefully Not Dying Girl.

"Good luck tomorrow, Mimi," she said.

They all chimed in: "We love you."

I closed the door after a last hug from Moe and went back to the kitchen. I cleaned up my burrito mess and took my last sips of water before beginning my twelve-hour fast. But as I opened the fridge to put the cheese away, I noticed that I had a lot of leftovers in there: withering French fries, Tupperware containers of decomposing pasta, and that appetizer I insisted we order at Olive Garden last week. For some reason their presence annoyed me, as if they were a burden on me. But really they'd be a burden on whoever needed to clean them out if I wasn't to return tomorrow.

I didn't have the energy to do dishes the night before the biggest day of my life. It was a trivial task, and by all definitions unnecessary. I also didn't want to take them from the fridge, because in some way they represented me. My name was scrawled on all the takeout boxes in crayon. The dishes were slathered in mozzarella cheese. Oddly, this was a very accurate depiction of *me*—tightly packed away in little plastic dishes, and slightly molding due to neglect.

A typhoon's worth of pressure built up in my chest at the idea of my mother throwing me into the trash can if I didn't make it out of the operating room. I nearly lost my shit looking at a pizza box. I knew I had to go to bed immediately. But I took out a piece of paper and pen instead and sat back down at the table. Alone and covered in burrito remains, I wrote the most dimwitted letter of all time. I hadn't planned on writing this letter, but the thought of leaving without saying anything to my family about the leftovers seemed ludicrous, so I had to do it.

Writing this letter was the single most terrifying thing I have ever done, and by far the stupidest. Scarier than first dates, trying exotic foods, and stand-up comedy. I laughed about it, then started to cry, then laughed at myself again. It's a good thing no one caught me writing it.

The letter was my last attempt to take myself seriously, which I was unable to do. But it wasn't about the leftovers or the goofy jokes to my dog. I wrote the letter because I was afraid of being forgotten. As ridiculous as it now sounds, I needed proof that I was there in that kitchen, saying goodbye. I wanted my story to be told, even on the back of a burrito-stained piece of paper—even if I didn't have much of a story to tell at the time. *The Girl Who Gets Sick and Leaves Messes Behind*. It would never have made it out of the screenwriter's room. Unlike *The Girl with the Dragon Tattoo*, it had no thrilling plot lines or character development. Just a short life and some dirty Tupperware.

After I wrote it I folded it into a small square, wrote "To Be Destroyed" on the front, and took it upstairs with me to stash semi-hidden by my bedside table. Just a casual death letter to my family on a Thursday evening. Then I crawled into bed, called my best friend Katrina, and melted into a puddle of sobs on my pillow.

"I am so scared," I cried. "What is going to happen to me tomorrow?"

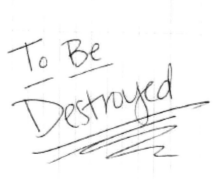

Dear Family,

If anyone finds this it means something bad happened ~~teety~~ today ... Woops.

I just want all of you to know that I love you so much and my time on this Earth has been pleasant because of you (wow, it's weird to actually write something like this.... I hope you don't ever have to read this...)

I know in my heart that we will be together again ... probably tomorrow, because you don't actually need to read this because I'm fine and I've already destroyed this letter and joked to you all about writing it.

This is ridiculous.

I'm going to bed. See you tomorrow, you'll never see this letter.

And Tucker: Stay Golden.

And sorry about all the leftovers I left in the fridge...

One more thing: I have a diary lying around somewhere ... happy hunting!

Love, M

Because *I didn't know.* This was the first moment I allowed myself to acknowledge how terrifying brain surgery would be. Now I considered for real that my end date could be tomorrow, October 3, 2014. I was horrified. I panicked. My last meal had been a frozen burrito, for fuck's sake.

"Everything will be okay," Kat said. "They're going to do the surgery, just like Dr. C said, and you will wake up and you will be fine."

This wasn't the first time someone had tried to convince me that I was okay. Obviously I wasn't. I have to wonder in what circumstances it is ever okay to leave a letter for your family to find after you die. How about never? Many months later, this letter would hurtle out of my notebook and onto my mother's lap as she sat on my bed with me. That was the least okay thing to happen in the history of not okay things.

I tried to grab the note from her hands.

"Let me read it!" She pulled the paper away and opened it. And I was fucked.

What happened next was rather traumatic. Mom read the letter and began to cry, and I tried to laugh my way out of the whole thing.

"Mom, it was a joke, okay? Just a ha-ha, funny joke! See?" I cracked a fake smile and waved the letter around her face like a theater prop.

Mom kept crying and I hugged her tightly, apologizing for being such an asshole and not burning the letter when I got home from the hospital. Actually, I'd forgotten about the letter entirely.

And no wonder. I don't recommend this type of letter writing to anyone. Looking death in the eye is not a hobby that we should take up between jobs like knitting or making tiny clay figurines. But writing the letter taught me that we truly only live once. No do-overs or repeats. There are no writer's rooms or director's cuts in the day-to-day scenes of our lives. We can't push the pause button and take a popcorn break.

Some people's lives end before they even begin; children are diagnosed with terminal cancer every day. Across the world men, women, and children are battling AIDS, Ebola, tuberculosis, strokes, heart attacks, domestic abuse, brain injuries, and gunshot wounds. And many of them don't make it to tell a recovery story.

So we tell it for them. Each of us carries bags filled with stories, folded up and sometimes forgotten until the opportune moment. Occasionally these traumas hurl themselves out of our hidden compartments and make a mess of our lives. Sometimes we wish they could be destroyed so that we didn't have to carry such a heavy bag of heartbreak around like an overstuffed grocery sack. But we carry them anyway.

We also carry love. Our friends go out of their way to make us smile and give us blankets and hugs and little Band-Aids for our hearts. Our mothers push nurses aside so that we can get the treatment we need. Our puppies love us when we are at our lowest of the low. And when we stop and take a moment to appreciate this love, our world is truly beautiful.

# Sit the Fuck Down, Helen

*Friday, October 3, 2014, 4:00 a.m.*

It is dark in my bedroom. I crack my eyes open to find the source of the sound. My alarm blares again from the window sill, forcing me out of bed, and I move with intention, each step careful, calculated. It's the morning of my surgery. My *brain* surgery.

They said to pack my bags for the weekend, so last night I collected clothes and facewash and toothpaste in a small purple backpack. I'm not sure why I needed to pack these things. I don't know how long I'll be gone. I don't know if I'll need them at all.

I shut off the alarm and waddle to the mirror to assess my current state. I look withered. My ribs poke out from my loose shirt. My hair is unruly as always, and I untangle the hair tie holding it all together. I'm thirsty this morning. But I'm not sure if I'm allowed to have water. I have to pee, but I'm not sure if I'm allowed to do that either. There are so many rules to the brain cutting, so many procedures that I tried to remember as they explained them over the phone yesterday.

The idea that someone will be opening my skull sickens me, so I ignore it.

I decide to take a shower. I decide to be clean. In a few hours everything will be messy, everything will be undone. I wash my hair slowly and run my fingers all over my head—no bumps, no pain. But I'm dizzy. I've been in the hot shower air too long, and the blood is rushing to my broken head. I shut off the water quickly and clear the soap from my eyes, then grasp the metal towel rack as I lift one foot out of the tub to dry ground. Any slip could be fatal, they said.

At a quarter to five I work my way down the stairs, holding the railing as if it will decide my future. It's quiet; Mom and Dad are still getting ready upstairs. Everyone is getting ready today. They're praying and hoping and holding on to the anxiety wrapped like tiny nooses around their necks.

Mom comes down the stairs. "Are you ready?" she asks.

"Yes," I say.

I say this even though it isn't true. The lie leaves my lips and fills the dimly lit kitchen. It bounces off the walls and echoes back to me and my little backpack. *You're not ready to die. I'm not ready to die.* I lied to my mom. I lied to my students. I am a fake and an actor and a fraud. I cannot tell any more jokes. So I get in the car.

The car ride to the hospital is quiet, but like the kitchen, it reverberates with the sound of my own deceit. I am en route. Mom points out a few buildings on the way—buildings from her youth, old apartments she lived in. She wants me to know. Maybe part of her thinks this will be the last time I'll make this drive, the last time I'll see these streets and buildings fly past my passenger window. I make sure to pay close attention.

~

When we got to the hospital, time sped up, everything swift and urgent. There was work to be done. I checked in to the surgery center, and Mom helped me take out my health insurance card and driver's license for the lady at the desk. They would hold on to these until after the surgery. I wanted to wonder why, but we had no time.

I sat in the small waiting room for only a few minutes. Across from me was an elderly couple sitting together, the old man holding the old woman's hand. Surgeries were things that old people had; it was normal for their bodies to break down and be fixed and re-fixed. I was an alien. I did not belong here.

My name was called, and my parents and I walked through the double doors for the pre-op procedures. They took my clothes from me. They took my shoes. They took my little purple bag. *You won't need these where you're going*, their eyes seemed to say.

In my paper gown, I sat awaiting instruction. First, I stumbled over to the weighing area and weighed in at a mere 109 pounds, almost 20 pounds lighter than my usual weight. Next was a urine sample. This was easy for me, as I hadn't gone since the night before. I urinated into the tiny cup and hoped that my disease would leave me too. *Just get out. I don't want to be here. It's not funny anymore.*

After placing the cup in a special compartment, I met with my anesthesiologist, who informed me that the possibility of my dying on the operating table was slim, but that I should sign this paperwork just in case. I was asked if I had a last will and testament and whether I would like to be resuscitated in the event that my heart stopped beating. *Yes, I would like to be resuscitated, thank you very fucking much*, I wanted to say. Instead, I signed on the dotted line. I did not read the fine print, nor did I want to. I didn't want to know what would happen to my little purple bag if I died on the table.

Then came the needles and IVs. I hadn't drunk any water in the past twelve hours, as instructed, and my veins were already invisible as it was. The first nurse searched with no success. She stabbed my arms twice on each side. Inside, my body was screaming, *Stop fucking poking me with needles*. But I was helpless. I couldn't scream. I'd probably just signed a paragraph in that fine print that forbade it.

After a second nurse and several more pokes, they brought in a young and handsome man with a pair of X-ray goggles. I wondered if he was my age and wanted to go on a quick date before my surgery. Maybe he'd steal some orange juice from the fridge, and we could hide out behind a curtain and pretend like none of this was happening. But it was happening. I couldn't make-believe myself out of this one.

The handsome nurse put on the X-ray binoculars and pinched my arms to find the veins. It hurt, and my arms were turning a shade of deep purple. I wanted to joke about it. I wanted to joke about the binoculars and my invisible veins. I wanted to joke about pissing in a cup and my ass hanging out of the back of my paper gown. But I couldn't. All I felt was queasy and numb.

I looked down to see that he had found the vein and injected me with some kind of fluid. That was probably in the small print of the paperwork too.

"You might feel it flush through you a little bit," he said.

It was strange. I did. I felt the tiny amount of fluid flow through me. I even tasted it. It was salty.

"Drink this, please," another nurse said. "It's for the nausea." She handed me a tiny black cup, and I threw it back like a shot of whiskey. It tasted like shit.

And then the pre-op procedures were over. Mom and Dad were still only inches away. A nurse placed a shiny gold operating cap on my head, and I asked her, wide-eyed, if I could keep this fancy hat. One last attempt at convincing myself that everything behind those mysterious doors would go according to plan.

"Absolutely," she said.

My next question seemed to disappear into the plastic curtains.

Mom and Dad grabbed for my hands and squeezed. "I love you," they said simultaneously.

The nurses wheeled my bed away, and our hands detached. I must have muttered that I loved them too. But I couldn't feel it anymore. My entire body was numb with fear. Everything was in slow motion. I could feel my heart trying to escape my chest, though, *thumpthumpthumpthumpthump*, like it was moving independently of the rest of my body.

The bed rolled through a set of heavy metal doors and into what resembled a movie set. Bright lights and shiny tools littered the room. I thought maybe there would be a camera nearby to catch my heart leaping out of my body. People moved around the room like extras in an action scene. They talked to each other as if I wasn't there. As if they were mid-take and running through their lines like normal. For them it was just another day at the office. I was smothered by anxiety. I was going to screw up my line.

I wondered if I would momentarily die on the table so that I could watch myself from the outside, floating above the table. I'd seen that in a movie once. I wondered if I would end up in a state of semi-afterlife in which I had to right my wrongs before being allowed into heaven. I thought about James and whether I could have changed our fate, if I could have kept us from exploding in such an epic manner. I pictured myself a ghost walking among the living, tracing my steps back to when I lost him. To when I lost myself. I thought about all the things I would say to him now, lying on this table under the florescent lights in my shiny gold cap and paper gown. I would tell him that it wasn't fair. That I was still angry at him. I would tell him that he'd regret everything, leaving me here on this table. But then I'd tell him that it wasn't his fault. I was on this table now because of *me*.

~

My eyes cracked open, and a nurse pulled a large yellow tube out of my throat.

"Shit," I panted. "Am I dead? Are you dead?"

A shrill, high-pitched beeping filled my eardrums, which I interpreted as a panic alarm. In my mind, I was waking up mid-surgery, and I wasn't supposed to. Something had gone horribly wrong.

A voice began talking to me from somewhere above my head. "We're both very much alive," the voice said, laughing. "Everything went fine." I didn't entirely believe the voice. I also couldn't see the voice. Something was off. I couldn't tell what it was.

My first two nurses, Sue and Ryan, I was told, wheeled me down to the anesthesia room, a precursor to the intensive care unit. I fluttered in and out of consciousness as florescent lights whizzed by me on the ceiling. Sue kept pestering me to stay awake, and Ryan spooned ice chips into my mouth upon request. I was so dehydrated that I asked him for ice chips every two seconds, opening my mouth like a baby bird waiting for Mommy's worm.

When you get out of a major surgery, before they take you to the ICU, you are brought to a special anesthesia room to sit with other patients who are also coming out of major surgeries. It's a room filled with drugged-up, half-conscious people who want their damn ice chips, goddamn it. I felt so marvelous from the drugs, I didn't want to go to the ICU now or ever. I just wanted to sleep in this little warm room.

Sue kept pinching me to stay awake. "How do you feel, Mimi?" she asked.

"Goooood. Real good." I slobbered onto my gown.

As I began opening my eyes for ten seconds at a time, I noticed that the nurses were playing a nasty prank on me and had flipped my bed on its side and strapped me to it. I was completely sideways, and I was pissed. Something had gone wrong in there.

"Real funny, Sue. Real funny."

"What's funny, Mimi?" She sounded genuinely confused.

"You're a real jokester, you know that? This was probably Ryan's idea, wasn't it?"

"What are you talking about?"

I told her.

"We didn't flip your bed on its side," she said. "Is that what you're seeing right now?"

My vision was not only double but also sideways. And quadruple. Everyone was horizontal. *What the fuuuuuuck, Sue.*

I wondered which parts of my brain they had tooled around with in there and whether I would ever see right side up again. *It would sure make for an interesting Ron Howard film*, I thought. I wasn't sure if this was actually funny or not, but I made a mental note to write it down later, assuming I still had fingers.

That's when fucking Helen showed up.

I closed my eyes again, ignoring Sue's pinches, trying to shake off the weirdness of my skewed vision. Then I heard yelling from the other side of the room.

"Helen! Sit down, Helen."

"Helen, could you please sit in the chair? *Helen*. Helen, please don't run over there."

"Helen, don't pull those out of your arms. Sit in the chair, Helen."

Helen's name was said at least a thousand times in the span of five minutes. Of course, I was so hopped up on drugs, it could have been thirty seconds—or thirty hours. I had no concept of time.

By now I could hear Helen causing an all-out ruckus around me, turning over chairs and shaking the curtains and IV bags.

I craned my stiff neck sideways to find one of my nurses. "Sue?"

"Yes, Mimi?"

"What the *fuck* is up with Helen?" I said with utmost seriousness.

Amid all the joking and the relief that I'd somehow survived a massive brain incision, I was exhausted. I wanted to sleep. I also wanted to not be seeing everything like I was a snow globe that someone had tipped onto its side. I didn't know Helen. I didn't know her story or what kind of surgery she'd survived or if something had gone wrong with her too. I didn't know if her coping mechanism was alcohol or cocaine or making jokes. I didn't know if she was in pain like I was. But I knew that I wanted her to shut the hell up.

Sue and Ryan burst into laughter. I felt deflated and embarrassed. Here I was, trying to relax and enjoy my drugs and ice chips post-surgery, and Helen was ruining everything. It sounded like every nurse in the hospital was chasing her around the room, trying to keep her from climbing the walls. *How ridiculously rude*, I thought. Didn't Helen know that the rest of us were in here too? I had to take matters into my own feeble hands.

I mustered the energy to lift my head and waved off Ryan as he offered me an ice chip. I tilted my head just barely, trying to find Helen in the room, and screeched at the top of my cracking voice: "Helen. Sit down. You got this, Helen. *Sit the fuck down.*" I collapsed back on the pillow pathetically but also heroically. I tried to start a round of applause, but I couldn't seem to accomplish more than a slow clap. Sue and Ryan were still laughing. Either my scolding had worked, or Helen didn't exist. It's entirely possible that she was a figment of my drugged-up imagination. I didn't exactly *see* her…but then again, I couldn't see anything.

When I arrived in the ICU to meet my parents, I was pissed off and had stories to tell. I told them about the yellow tube in my throat and the nice ice chips. I told them I couldn't see straight. I asked them if they had seen Helen anywhere and to put a Kick Me sign on her back if they saw her roaming the halls, tearing down shit.

I was still steaming with anger when Sue and Ryan handed me off to Deana, my first ICU nurse. Deana liked me immediately, probably because she'd heard gossip that I'd yelled at an imaginary woman named Helen who was supposedly running around the anesthesia room, destroying my life.

I rested in my new ICU room as unknown substances pulsed through my veins, making me lose track of the stitches in my head. I sipped water and tried to forget Helen's screams and the bright lights of the operating room. Mom stroked my hand, even though it was covered in IV wires. I was too tired to feel lucky to be alive. But at least Helen had shut the fuck up.

# I'm Peeing as We Speak

"Mom?" I cracked my eyes open to locate her shapes. Immediately after my surgery they'd hauled me into another MRI like a sack of potatoes to make sure they'd done the surgery correctly. I sure didn't think so. My vision was double *and* sideways, everything just shapes and pigments. I was in the intensive care unit now, or at least so I'd been told.

"Right here, sweetie," she said. "Do you need something?"

"Yeah," I said. "I need to pee."

"You already are."

"I'm sorry, what?" *Like hell I am*, I thought. If another nurse had dumped a bag of IV fluid in my lap, I was going to stage a mutiny.

"They put in a catheter while you were under," she said.

I shuffled my blankets and peeled back my cotton hospital gown. Even my wonky eyes could make out a small tube coming out of my lady bits.

"What the fuck is this?" I was tempted to yank it out right then and there.

"Leave it in, sweetheart," she said. "It's so you don't have to get out of bed to go to the bathroom."

"Where exactly does this tube go?"

"The bucket under your bed."

I cringed at that. Somebody was paid for this. To help me pee in a bucket. And I was unconscious when it all went down, not that I'd have wanted to be awake for this procedure. But I would have liked to know about the piss bucket situation ahead of time.

I'd lost all modesty. There was no way around it. I was peeing into a bucket on the floor as I lay pathetically on my side, trying to make the ceiling tiles stop spinning. Privacy had gone out the window alongside my sanity. Parts of my body that even I didn't like to see, other people had seen in detail. And lots of people. Doctors, nurses, physical therapists, and interns could simply tell me to drop trou and I had to obey. Perfect strangers removed tubes from my Bermuda Triangle, helped me scrub my armpits, and performed other arduous tasks that no human should have to do for another human. The number of people who had seen me naked had more than quadrupled in a matter of minutes.

I'd relieved myself in front of people before. That's what you did at frat parties when you were too drunk to make it in there on your own. I'd had some of my deepest conversations sitting on a toilet while my improv sisters perched on the counters, checking their hair and makeup. But this was something else entirely. I'd just woken up from brain surgery, and IVs were sticking out of my arms like tangled spaghetti noodles. I couldn't move my head or most of my body. I wanted to go home, or at least be able to get to the bathroom on my own. But instead of confronting these fears, what did I do? I joked about it, you guys.

I decided after the initial discovery of the catheter that it was a funny thing, a joke that should be shared. In my infinite wisdom, thanks to veins full of new painkillers, I pointed the catheter out to everyone who came within earshot. Friends, nurses, stuffed animals—everyone.

"Hello, Auntie Karen! Yes, I'm doing fine—but have you *seen* my secret toilet device?" I'd say.

Two of my friends were the hardest hit by my antics. Heather and Katie, from my college improv team, were used to joking around with me. We'd spend hours in the bowels of the art building, coming up with new team names, practicing our bits, and tricking nearby art students into coming inside the auditorium to see our shows. But no amount of improv training could prepare them for the piss bucket.

"We brought you some donuts—" Heather said.

"Wash your hands!" Mom shouted at them as they entered the room. Anyone who came near me in the ICU had to disinfect themselves. I was starting to think that my brain bleed was contagious.

"Hey, you guys!" I said, my head crooked on the pillow. "Come on in. Check this out…"

I told them about my catheter, Helen, and when I predicted my brain drugs would wear off again. Their faces displayed utter shock. The last time they'd seen me, I was probably running around a stage, telling my fellow improvisers to stop asking questions and to make stronger character choices. Now I was a lopsided little sick girl bragging about my own excrement.

Despite my new horrific reality, Heather and Katie handled it well. They saw the real me: the me in this moment, unable to lift my head or body, drinking from a hospital sippy cup and trying to laugh about my screwed-up vision. This must have scared the shit out of them. And yet here they were in the ICU, doing bits with me about the *special potty.*

Once I could move enough to get to the bathroom with help from the nurses, the device came out, uncomfortably, I might add. But I didn't gain any more privacy in the process. Instead of the bucket, now I had a team of nurses who demanded that they walk me to the toilet, sit me down, and watch me as I went to the bathroom. This didn't go over well with me. So I tried to sneak in a quick pee break like a ninja when the nurses were switching shifts.

It turned out that walking the three feet to the toilet and sitting myself down was a task newly difficult and challenging. I reluctantly used a walker at a snail's pace, and when I tried to get my underwear down, I nearly ate shit on the floor. I was too dizzy and unstable to do this alone.

I hadn't realized how much of a child I'd feel after being told I couldn't go to the bathroom on my own. They didn't trust me with this task. They didn't trust me with anything. I suspect someone would even have forced a spoon of oatmeal down my throat if I hadn't felt like eating that day. *Choo choooo, here comes the train, Mimi! Two more bites, then we'll go to the potty!* Everything post-surgery seemed ridiculous. Was this something old people in nursing homes thought about daily?

Despite all my attempts at joking, the first twenty-four hours in the ICU were terrifying. I'd awoken from what felt like a dream and arrived to a nightmare. My body operated in strange ways now, and it had rules—rules covering what I could and couldn't do on my own with this new self. There were medications I had to take and needles to be stuck in the crooks of my arms. Everything required a team of trained nurses or qualified professionals. My life ceased to feel like my own in that room; I was simply an item that must be maintained in stable condition. I had an identification number and a brightly colored bracelet with my name, date of birth, and hospital room number printed on it. The bracelet had a bar code that was scanned with every new blood draw or dose of medication. Each morning they would take inventory of me like I was a Scandinavian-named piece of furniture at IKEA.

The hallway was loud, I noticed. People were constantly running about and shouting. I could hear ambulances zooming from the street to a garage at the front. And at night the ICU became nightmare central. I couldn't sleep through the sounds of screaming and pain from the rooms next to me. The lights in the hall were always on, and shadows of frantic nurses and doctors scurried across my squinted eyelids. I clenched my eyes closed tighter, but my body couldn't ignore the symphony of human anguish surrounding me.

But even in that harsh environment, my mother still found ways to make me comfortable. I was cleared to take my first shower with a nurse, and she stepped in.

I tried to shrug off her attempts to help remove my clothes, but my T-shirt ended up stuck over my head. I sat pathetically on the side of my hospital bed and awaited rescue.

"It's okay, baby," she said softly. "Let me help you."

Mom helped my fragile, naked body into the shower chair and removed my hair tie. As she massaged shampoo gently into my scalp, locks of hair fell to the shower drain.

"It's supposed to be the other way around." I chuckle-sobbed as she rinsed my head, making sure to move slowly over the wound. "I'm supposed to do this for *you* when you get old."

The water felt so good on my head.

"I know, I know," she cooed. "It's okay."

Large clumps of hair fell out of my ponytail and to the shower floor.

I'd needed the surgery to fix me. But had it really? Had the new MRIs revealed a renewed sense of self? A real-life purpose that didn't revolve around fantasy and make-believe? Could these metal donuts and piss buckets reflect back my future? I doubted they could change me from within, change the deeply rooted wires that had tangled me up in a farce for years.

There were parts of me that didn't work right—eyes that couldn't see straight or singular and limbs that wouldn't respond—and now locks of hair were falling out. Mom soothed me and told me that all these things were temporary. I still wasn't convinced. Deep down I was worried that I was beyond repair; that this helplessness was my new reality.

I didn't know it then, but Mom was holding back quiet tears the entire time.

# The Only Hepburn I Ever Hated

This chapter is not about Katharine or Audrey Hepburn, both of whom I quite enjoy. This is also not the chapter where I run away in Rome to escape my identity as a European princess and meet Gregory Peck.

Unfortunately my time in the ICU was far less classy than my mentioning these film stars might have had you believe. There were no devilishly handsome male nurses or opportunities to sneak out a window and into the busy streets of Italy. It was just a lot of me getting stabbed with needles.

I survived my first scary night in the ICU, but during the day the place was just as terrifying. I was under constant watch. The beds beeped loudly if I tried to get out of them, like I was trying to hop barbed wire. Nurses rotated shifts as though they were monitoring a prisoner of war. They brought me food and changed out my water bag, at least, so I felt like they were following POW ethical codes. Until Deana came in that morning with the world's most alarming announcement.

"All right, Mimi." Her smile was skewed because I was still seeing the world at a 45-degree angle. "Here's your pepper shot—"

"Whaaa…" I muttered in drugged-out confusion. Before I had time to react, Deana had lifted my cotton gown and stabbed me square in the stomach with a needle.

From my side view, I'd thought that Deana seemed nice. Her voice was kind, and while her face was mostly a blur, her hair was pleasant enough. She'd asked me about my life, my teaching, and how I'd ended up in this crummy ICU bed. But then she stabbed me with the needle, and I had to wonder which Russian mobster had sent her to kill me for my misbehavior. The needle burned in my stomach for ten minutes as I shouted choice words at Deana in between moaning and rubbing my sore and bloated tummy. "Deana, if that is your real name, I thought I could trust you! I thought we had a mutual love of geography! *Who sent you?*"

I was still too drugged up to connect the dots, so when the pain subsided, I shrugged it off as some strange but legitimate medical procedure that I'd agreed to in the fine print of all that paperwork. I ordered a new ice baggy by pressing the button on the bed, summoning Deana. It was like magic.

"Hi, Mimi, what can I do for you?" she said.

"I'll take three filets mignons with a baked potato on the side and some lightly grilled asparagus...Oh, and can you load up that baked potato? Let's not play around here, I'm a grown-up. I need that potato smothered in everything...I'm just kidding. I need a new ice baggy."

"Sure thing, Mimi. And that reminds me, I'll be right back," she said, and left the room.

When she returned, I fantasized that maybe she'd brought the filet mignon. It was miles away in a dark freezer at my parents' house, but it haunted my dreams.

"Time for your Hepburn shot!" She smiled.

I tried to brace for impact, but it was too late; the pain from the needle shot up my stomach.

"Deana, stop that!" I yelled.

The anesthesia was wearing off now. Still, I didn't realize until the third stabbing that what Deana was giving me was a heparin injection. It was finally explained to me that the heparin shot was a blood thinner being used to prevent clots.

The idea that Deana was trying to change the consistency of my blood only reaffirmed my belief that she was secretly a hitman. I was confined to a bed and could hardly move. Couldn't my blood move around in there without the stabbing?

I'm that person who might faint even talking about a needle. The very thought of the human body sends my brain into complete shutdown mode. Blood draws are hilarious. I collapse on the floor, and nurses hand me cute little juice cups to bring me back to consciousness. I'm a complete joke.

While I would not wish this needly torture on anyone, I certainly felt rugged and awesome when I found I could just roll with it after my brain surgery. *Hey, they're about to stab me with a needle. Look away if it grosses you out. Doesn't bother me one bit. Look at all these pokes in my belly! I'm a human pincushion!* After several days in the ICU, I acquired quite the impressive bruise collection. But I was at peace with my body becoming a shoddy recreation of *Starry Night*, because it proved how tough I was. I wore my bruises with honor while also whining when my siblings poked at them and asked me if they hurt. Yes, they hurt. Why do people do that?

The funniest thing about this was that I'd go in for a routine eye exam many months later, and my rough-and-tough alter ego would make a hasty exit. I passed out in the examination chair after being asked for my allergies and a brief medical history. I awoke in a haze with six nurses on me like a white girl at Starbucks during Pumpkin Spice Latte season. They were placing cold towels on my head and feeding me juice through a straw. They have good juice there, you know. One nurse stayed with me to make sure I didn't relapse into hilarious unconsciousness. I reassured her that this was kind of my thing.

Deana was gentler and kinder than I originally believed, what with all the heparin shots. She made an otherwise scary place feel more comfortable for me. Her words were soft and caring, and I never went a single minute without a fresh ice baggy for my pounding head. She was the sort of person you don't believe exists, because she was that self-sacrificing.

We were cosmically destined to have met each other, because Deana was intertwined in my fate and my future beyond the ICU. But I was still loopy from the drugs, lights, and sounds; I didn't know it yet.

# There's No Crying in Rehab

You know that scene from *A League of Their Own*? The one where…wait. Maybe you haven't seen it yet. Okay, stop right now and troll around the internet or your nearest Blockbuster turned hipster bar and grab this movie and watch it. Right now.

Are you back? Great. Wasn't that just the feel-good movie you were looking for? You're welcome.

Let's try this again. *Now* do you remember that scene where Tom Hanks gets mad at the blondie for something silly she did on the field, and she starts crying? Then Hanks is all like, "There's no crying in baseball!" It's a great cinematic moment in our nation's history, and I hope that you appreciate it as much as I do.

We'll get to why this scene is important in a minute.

No, we weren't going to a baseball game. But after what seemed like an eternity spent in the hospital, escaping to anywhere else would have been a godsend. Loud beeping, flashing lights, and yelling down the hallway had kept me up at night for hours. Hospital food disgusted me, and I longed for my lumpy, crappy bed and furniture hog of a puppy. I'd peed into a bucket and was over it. I missed taking showers by myself. And I'm sure Helen was just having a fucking ball next door.

After I stabilized, I was admitted to Saint Joseph Hospital for a night. In the morning a doctor came in with a clipboard and a pair of glasses balanced loosely on his nose. "Ready to go home, kiddo?"

I hated being called *kiddo*. Of course this kiddo was ready to go home, sir. This kiddo was a grown-ass woman and could drive herself home—oh, wait, scratch that. *I can't see straight. And I think the bones in my legs are smaller than they were before this, because now I need assistance getting out of bed. Did I mention that I can't hold my head up straight? That it feels like somebody took an ice pick to my skull? Can I get some more Percocet? On second thought, I don't think the kiddo is ready to go home.*

When the doctor asked me the question, my mother shot death glares at his droopy glasses. She couldn't voice it then in my tiny hospital room, but she was scared to death. I was just stoked to be feeling like Al Pacino in *Scarface*, with my long list of narcotics.

Before I was sent on my merry way, some therapists dropped in to check on the status of the kiddo. A tiny Asian man with what I thought were square spectacles came in and introduced himself. He had a name, I'm sure. I'm gonna call him Phil. I didn't write down Phil's real name, because I was too busy trying to update social media with a witty post-surgery status. "Surgery went fine, y'all. Seeing double is super interesting, and I get all the pain meds that I want," I tweeted.

Mr. Physical Therapist Man Phil and I went on a stroll around the nurses' station. And when I say *stroll*, I mean that a team of nurses had to hoist me out of bed with a gait belt, and it took me about ten minutes to shuffle three feet with a walker.

"Look at her moving," he said in delight. "She's ready to walk right out of this joint!"

Walking the three feet had exhausted me. Putting one foot in front of the other was hard before surgery, but now it seemed impossible. I waddled back into the room and collapsed onto the bed to await my next batch of Percocet. I hadn't shit in days and I saw two of everything constantly now, but at least I had on-demand access to fun drugs. I wondered if I'd still have my 24/7 Percocet hookup if they kicked me out of this place. That could be a serious problem.

An occupational therapist, a slender woman with her hair tucked back in a neat ponytail, had seen the whole thing. She watched me roll over in the bed, moaning, and turned to the other therapist.

"She's twenty-two, Phil," she said to Fake Phil. "Not eighty-five. She should be sprinting around that nurses' station. I want a second opinion."

That got me worried again. What if the surgery hadn't been a smash out of the park like Dr. Crawford promised? Having to get a second opinion about my current state didn't thrill me, but I agreed I might need more professional insight than that of my buffoon of a therapist. *Maybe he should go on a date with my old friend Dr. Pollock, I thought. Doc Pollock and Fake Phil hit the town—sounds like a match made in asshole heaven.*

The occupational therapist, we'll call her Savior Sally, called a second physical therapist to assess me. This therapist had me walk in a straight line next to a wall in the hallway and perform several balancing exercises that made me look like the drunkest bitch at the party. My movements were slow and sloppy, just like when I used to pretend I liked tequila shots in college. And just like in college, I was in a weird, drunk blur, grasping at the wall haphazardly as someone held me up while I protested, "No. I got dis! Really, no srsLyy, I can dO ett by m'selF!"

Savior Sally told Fake Phil that this kiddo was not ready to go home. Not even a little bit. She advised that I be sent to a place called Spalding Rehabilitation Center for intensive physical, occupational, and speech therapy. It wasn't covered under our insurance plan, but Savior Sally didn't give a shit, because it was the rehab that I needed. Sally was probably the only person my mother *didn't* want to punch in the face that morning.

"Spalding is the best facility that we have here," she said. "It's in Aurora, so you will be close enough to visit her while she undergoes treatment. I highly recommend we get her into Spalding as soon as possible and let your insurance deal with the rest later."

Mom's face was glowing with hope for the kiddo. I, on the other hand, was blissfully ignorant and on a shitload of Percocet.

We arranged to move me over to Spalding the next morning. My mother opted for the hospital transportation services to deliver me from the hospital to rehab.

"I'm okay, Mom," I said. "I can just ride with you." I didn't need a fancy hybrid ambulance van. I packed up my stained clothing and tried to untie my balloon from the foot of the bed with my bumbling fingers. I dizzily reached for my backpack, where I'd stashed some chocolate, and the room began beeping. I'd set off the motion sensors in the bed, which informed the entire hallway that I was up to no good.

"No," Mom said. "The minute we turn down medical services, they are no longer liable for your safety."

"My *safety*?" If I could have, I would have done a double-take. "Mom, my head is hanging off my neck right now."

I was itching pretty bad to get out of there, though. I'd never been to a rehabilitation center, but I hoped that it would be like Grammy's assisted living center. Before she passed, we'd often visit her apartment-style hospital setup. It still had nurses and doctors and pressure cuffs, but she had her own comfy bed and a small kitchenette and sitting area. If memory serves me, she might have even had a little Keurig machine in there. She had the hookup. I prayed that I'd have a Keurig in my rehab room too.

I longed for a cup of coffee. I also wondered what kind of people I would meet in rehab. Maybe I'd find a cute brain-damaged NHL player. Maybe our wheelchairs would get twisted up in the hallway before breakfast. *Maybe* we'd fall in love over our mutual love of puppies and *How I Met Your Mother*.

A mystery van pulled up to the curb and hauled me from my fictional rehab love affair. Mom followed, looking frazzled. The side door opened to reveal a gigantic ramp, and a friendly man rolled my wheelchair onto it and pushed a button, sending me and my little chair off the ground and into the van like I was boarding a spaceship. He crawled in after me and strapped my wheels into the car.

Mom gave me a worried look. She got in her car and followed us over with the backseat full of the baked goodies and flower pots people had sent me.

I don't recall most of the drive, but it was bumpy and painful. I'm not a doctor or anything, but I would have given the kiddo a fucking neck brace. As my head wandered aimlessly, looking for a place to reside, I began a pleasant conversation with my chauffeur. Was his name David? Brian? I don't know, I'd just gotten out of brain surgery, for crying out loud. He was nice.

"How long have you been driving people around in this fancy spaceship?" I asked.

"Couple years now," he said. "You comfy back there?"

After a twenty-minute drive, we pulled into the parking lot of Spalding Rehabilitation Center. David/Brian rolled me into the brightly lit lobby as Mom came hurtling through the double doors.

We checked in at the front desk and were instructed to go to the second floor to room 235 and await instructions. Dad met us in the lobby and pushed my wheelchair into the elevator. He wouldn't be popping any wheelies today.

David/Brian waved as the elevator doors closed. "Good luck, Mimi!" he said.

We rolled along the second-floor hallway like this was a slow-motion scene in a movie again. Nurses and staff smiled at me as we passed by. Strange health advice posters lined the walls like missing person ads. We rolled by the dining hall, and I caught a glimpse of stacks of blue and yellow trays. The doors to a gymnasium cracked open to reveal old people on exercise bicycles and passing medicine balls to each other. If the ambulance van was a spaceship, then I certainly had landed on the moon.

We arrived at room 235. The door was already open.

"This must be it," Mom said. "Your new home."

"My *what*?" I glared anxiously at a pressure cuff dangling from the wall.

"It's just for a little while, sweetie," Dad said.

The walls were painfully white, and the florescent lights hurt my eyes. On the wall was a wastebasket for needles. I looked to the bed—a hospital bed, with buttons. It was probably motion activated, and alarms would blare if I moved off it. This was familiar now.

A door immediately to the right revealed a bathroom and shower. The toilet had a tiny plastic bin resting inside, to collect my nonexistent shit. The shower had no doors or steps or enclosures; the entire bathroom *was* the shower. A panic button hung above the shower faucet.

Outside the windows I could see the slowly turning leaves of fall. I crawled out of the wheelchair and onto the stiff bed. I curled myself into a mooshy ball and sobbed.

I looked around the room and cried and cried. Mom crawled into the tiny bed too and cradled me. Dad held my hand, and I shifted from my fetal position to make eye contact with them both.

"There's no crying in rehab." I sniffled, feeling like the wimpiest Hanks ever.

Mom, Dad, and I laugh-cried in room 235 until a nurse came to give us the rundown of what Spalding Rehab would be like:

*Three hours of physical, occupational, and speech therapy each day. Breakfast is at seven thirty. Lunch at noon. Dinner at five. No coffee. No Keurigs. Visiting hours are seven in the morning until nine at night daily. Outside food is fine; you just can't leave. Use the call button on your bed for nursing assistance. Put this Q-tip in your mouth and then into this test tube. You will be under quarantine your first few days.*

*Quarantine?* The whole thing sounded insane. But this was my new home now. And Hanks wasn't here to tell me not to cry.

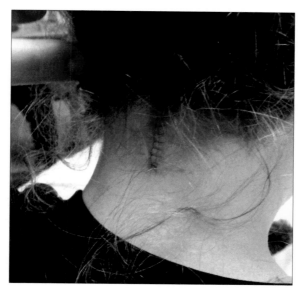

*There's nothing sexier than discovering that your brain surgeon can stitch in a straight line.*

## The Broomstick Test

In the morning I learned the ropes. And by that, I mean dangled from them helplessly. I'd tossed and turned all night. Spalding wasn't nearly as terrifying as the ICU, but I still heard the familiar buzz of doors opening and closing or nurses moving about the rooms so they could stab us all with needles. I wasn't allowed to leave my room due to the mysterious quarantine rule, so my breakfast was brought to me with a bright "Hello! Welcome to Spalding!"

I sleepily tossed a few spoonfuls of egg into my mouth and rolled over. I still couldn't taste. The left side of my tongue was performing a protest and refused to work. My body ached too, like someone had rammed the back of my neck with a pickup truck. I searched for the right place for my neck to not slide off the pillow.

Just when I'd readjusted myself in the stiff white sheets, a different woman entered my room, a black woman in her forties. I mustered the strength to roll over to meet her eyes, my stomach lurching as though I'd dropped from the top of a roller coaster. I wondered if this seasickness would ever subside. All that ill-prescribed Dramamine from a few months before could have come in handy now.

I peered at her multiple shadows. This was some real *Twilight Zone* kind of shit. "Deana?" I asked. "Is that you?" It was her; it had to be. I was sure she had a needle ready to stab my squishy tummy. I thought I was hallucinating.

"Hi, Mimi. I'm Vicki, your physical therapist," she said softly, then raised her eyebrows at me. "Wait, did you say Deana?"

I nodded. With my double vision, I could have sworn she looked exactly like my friend Deana down in the ICU.

"Deana is my sister's name," she said. "Do you know her?"

"Deana took care of me in the ICU," I said. "She stabbed me with a lot of needles, but she was cool."

"Oh my goodness, she's never going to believe this!" She smiled. "I'm going to have to call her tonight and tell her that you're here!"

It excited me that the world was so small and intimate. My time at Spalding would now be a family affair. Through every small success and utter failure I'd encounter, Vicki and Deana would be part of it with me.

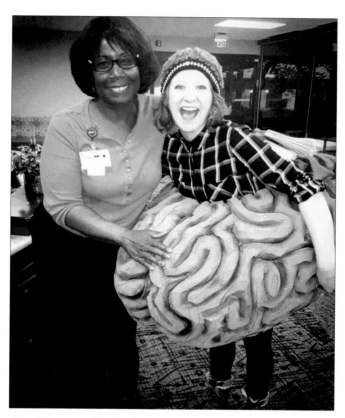

*The famous Vicki, also known on the second floor as Attila the Hun for her aggressive physical therapy tactics.*

Before we could go to the gym facility for my first physical therapy lesson, Vicki needed to outfit me in some gear. She brought in a wheelchair and locked it at the foot of the bed. "See how it doesn't move on you like that?" Vicki held out her arms to guide me into the chair. "Always remember to lock your wheelchair."

*What a fucking dumb rule*, I thought. *I don't even need a wheelchair.* Then I looked at my legs and remembered that I'd needed help using them the night before to go pee. Apparently I needed assistance getting into the wheelchair too. I needed help getting to the help chair.

The brain surgery was supposed to fix these mobility issues. But it hadn't.

Vicki helped my arms through a yellow paper smock and tied it tightly behind my back like a straitjacket. Then she guided my fumbling hands into a pair of blue gloves and placed a yellow face mask over my nose and mouth, tucking the straps behind my ears. Lastly she took a thick pink belt from the wall and tied it around my waist securely.

"I look like Walter from *Breaking Bad*," I said. "What's all this for?"

"Your MRSA swab test hasn't come through yet," she said. "We have to make sure you pass that test so that we know you are healthy; otherwise you'd get the other patients sick."

"Well, I'm obviously not healthy, Vicki," I said. "This we know for sure." I settled my suited-up body back into the wheelchair. But I didn't have time to focus on the discomfort of the disease prevention wardrobe; there was work to be done.

The first exercise Vicki introduced me to was walking over an arrangement of sticks in a pattern:

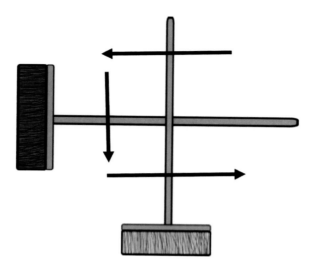

In other words, walking over broomsticks.

I felt ridiculous. Just weeks ago I'd been training for my half marathon and buying cute teacher outfits and unreasonably high heels to teach in. Now a stranger in a brain hospital was telling me to walk over broomsticks? Nothing added up.

"This is my therapy?"

"Yep," Vicki said. "I want you to walk in a C pattern once and back again as fast as you can without hurting yourself."

She locked my wheelchair in front of a pile of sticks, then assembled them into a T shape.

"The standard time for this task is about eight seconds," she said. "When you're ready, I can help you up." I nodded, and she hoisted me to a standing position.

I readjusted my face mask and tried to move toward the sticks. My feet were like rebellious teenagers. They slugged along and made tiny movements. *Move it along, damn you.* Vicki was still holding me up with the pink belt as we inched closer to the sticks.

"Are you ready?"

"Yeah." I breathed heavily. "You can let go now."

The moment her fingers left the belt, I was in a free fall. My body couldn't find solid footing. Vicki grasped the belt, and I stood up straight again.

"I'm right here, okay? I'm going to start the timer." I'd forgotten that this was a timed exercise. It felt like hours since I'd left the wheelchair beside me. Seconds became minutes and hours in the gym; time slogged by alongside my sleepy teenager feet. I stumbled onto the sticks, Vicki holding me up the entire time. We moved slowly in the *C* pattern as broomsticks lurched out at me at every step. My eyes saw them multiply before me, each one targeting my toes and trying to trip me up.

Finally I completed the pattern, and Vicki guided me carefully back to the locked wheelchair. I was panting beneath my face mask, and my hands were sweaty under the plastic gloves. My hair was clumped up under my mask. I felt sticky and wrong. I never wanted to do this broomstick bullshit again.

"How did I do?" I wheezed and leaned back in the chair.

"Fifty-two seconds," Vicki said.

The task took me fifty-two seconds. *Fifty-two*. It normally took eight. On a teacher grading scale, that was a giant fucking failure. I dropped my head in defeat and allowed my hair to fall helplessly into my face. How was it that in two months I had lost the ability to work my legs properly and see straight? How could something so simple be so fucking hard? I was dumbfounded and embarrassed. What was worse was that Vicki had held me up the entire time. She'd assisted me, and still I'd failed. What would this have looked like had she not been beside me? Would I have tripped and cracked my head open right there on the cold tile?

I wanted to cry. I wanted to scream into my face mask and curse my stupid body. Walking over a stick was the easiest thing I could think of to do, yet I'd failed at it. I didn't see how I'd ever be able to go back home. I couldn't imagine something vaguely resembling the life I lived before these broomsticks made me question everything.

I bit my quivering lip and allowed Vicki to roll me and my needed wheelchair to my next session: occupational therapy with Jamie.

Jamie had red hair and a kind face. Her eyes glowed green, and she kneeled in front of my wheelchair and took my hands in hers. "I'm excited to work with you," she said. That made no sense to me, considering the shit I'd pulled a moment ago.

"Before we get started today, I just want you to know that you're brave," she said as a lump formed in my weak throat. "I've heard about your journey getting here and dealing with doctors and people who wouldn't take your injury seriously. I've heard how amazing you've been dealing with this—"

"I'm not, though." I started to whimper. "I'm not brave."

"You are, Mimi. You have been fighting for your life."

I sobbed in total denial. I was weak and brittle, like an injured bird. How could this stranger see strength where there was none? Didn't she know it had just taken me fifty-two seconds to take one step over a broomstick? Couldn't she see that I was still heartbroken over a boy who'd left me stranded in a parking lot for another woman? Did she even know about the piss bucket fiasco?

Jamie handed me some tissues, and I blew my dripping nose loudly. This was only my first day in rehab, and I was already coming unglued. I knew that being in this strange place would help me; I didn't know how, though. I wanted to be strong yet denied the fact that I already was. What was clear to me now was that I was disabled. There could be no more joking around it; my legs didn't work, my eyes were screwed up, and I was tired of eating food I couldn't taste. I'd underestimated how bodies worked and didn't work. I couldn't just be along for the ride. I needed to reassemble the ride after a severe technical catastrophe had derailed the entire thing.

Jamie allowed me time to compose myself, and then she rolled me to a table covered in plastic medicine bottles. My task was to open as many bottles as possible. With my left hand. The one that didn't work.

"You want me to do what now?" I asked, readjusting my glasses as my head drifted half off my neck.

"Give it a try," Jamie said. "As many as you can in thirty seconds. Go!"

I'd opened thousands of medicine bottles in my life. I'd turned a thousand door handles, and I'd probably walked over broomsticks just fine. But now Jamie was asking the impossible. I picked up a small orange tube and grasped the cap. *Righty tighty, lefty loosey.* I tugged at the cap and tried to twist it. It wasn't coming off. Apparently they'd fucked around with the part of my brain responsible for the simplest of tasks. I wanted to cry again, looking down at my stupid hands fighting to get the cap off, but I worried they'd think all the crying was weird and send me down to the *other* hospital. Of course, thinking I was crazy for wanting to cry was completely crazy in itself. My emotional capacity was right on point for the intensity of my injury and had been described to me as a side effect that could decrease over time. But I'd always been an emotional person. What if this was my new reality? Crying over broomsticks and bottle caps?

After much panting and lightheadedness I finally popped it off. "I did it!" I screamed.

"I knew you could do it!" Jamie cheered, and I felt like I'd crossed the finish line at my half marathon.

We sat with the medicine bottles for twenty more minutes, me twisting and contorting my hands to pop the caps off. It was demanding work; I literally had to tell my hands what to do, because they didn't know how. Slowly my neurons were linking together what my brain wanted to do and what my hands were capable of doing. By the end I'd opened approximately fifteen bottles of various shapes and sizes. It felt like the biggest success I'd ever had—bigger than any teaching high I could imagine, more of a rush than I'd ever had from running. Jamie high-fived me cautiously.

"Wonderful job, Mimi," she said. "Now you get an hour break, and then Kendra will come get you for speech."

I didn't know what kind of speech I was supposed to be making, but I was happy to have a break. Jamie wheeled me back to my room, where a nurse was waiting to take off my medical gear and help me back into bed. I collapsed under the covers and fell asleep within minutes. I never knew I could be so tired from broomsticks and bottle caps.

~

I don't remember my dreams, but I'm sure they were lovely and involved no wheelchairs or broomsticks or IV baggies. Then suddenly my nap was over, and a shorter, friendly-looking woman sat at my bedside speaking to me.

"Hello, Mimi," she said. "It's time to wake up. My name is Kendra, and I'm here for your speech therapy."

I wrestled myself up to a seated position and reached out one weak hand to shake hers. "Hi," I said. "Sorry, I was so tired after the other therapy this morning."

"Understandable. Let's get started, and then they can bring you some lunch when we're done! You don't need to go anywhere; we can stay in here today."

The idea of lunch excited me, even though I knew I wouldn't taste much, so I rubbed the goo out of my eyes and sat up straighter.

Kendra unpacked a large bag and placed several books on my skinny side table. She got out a notepad. "Today we're going to do some tests on your memory and executive functioning," she said. I'd only heard that term once before in a high school psychology class. As far as I could recall, it was a job the brain did that allowed people to get something done without becoming distracted.

Kendra opened one of the books and asked me to identify the pictures on the pages: cars, houses, shoes, forks, and common household items. I flashed back to sitting in Mrs. Ruffalo's K3 classroom, frustrated as hell. She made us sing along to the alphabet song, using laminated placards, every single day for three years. By the third grade I was full of pent-up rage that the letter *A* always had to stand for *apple* and not some other interesting word like *abstract* or *adventure*. I wanted to write a book about a cat named Tibbs. I wanted to build nests for birds outside, made of grass and pebbles. Not do this stupid alphabet bullshit. I had that on lock.

When Kendra showed me the pictures, I flew through them.

"Couch."

"Hose."

"Dog."

"Wheel."

I shouted them out one after another. I was a picture-matching rock star. Until I came across one image.

"That's a…" I stared at it long and hard. "This is ridiculous," I said, bubbling with panic. Just seconds ago I'd been cocky. Now I couldn't recognize the easiest thing in the world.

"Do you know what this picture is?" Kendra asked.

"Of course I do, I just…can't, um…"

"I'll give you a hint," she said. "It's used for taking pictures."

I knew that. I knew exactly what it was. James was a photographer. We'd brought one of these on our trip to Paris so that we could take pictures of the Eiffel Tower.

"Is it an art thingy?" I asked, even though I knew that was the wrong answer. "Like you put art on top of it to paint it?"

"An art easel?"

"Yeah, is it an art easel?"

"This is not an art easel," she said. "This is a camera tripod."

Of course it was. I'd completely blanked. *Tripod.* I rolled the word over my tongue. *T-r-i-p-o-d.* It sounded like a new word, one I'd only now discovered. It was the strangest thing, other than tripping over broomsticks and taking twenty minutes to open a medicine bottle.

I hadn't been prepared for how hard rehab would be. The friendly van driver had rolled me through the double doors of what I imagined would be a day spa, for fuck's sake. I'd expected to be able to heal my body at lightning speed, and with little effort on my part. I knew nothing of therapy techniques or that there were even different kinds of therapy I'd have to do in order to retrain my brain. I hadn't even thought my brain was trainable; it simply sat in my head and performed tasks without my knowledge of its function. It was like a computer; obviously it was hard at work sending emails and bits of information at top speeds across continents and bouncing off satellites, but I didn't have a clue how it worked in there.

And soon I would be asking it to do more things both familiar and strange, foreign, impossible. Kendra would add numbers to my word problems, Vicki would add balance boards, and Jamie would introduce Excel spreadsheets and recipes. This would without a doubt be the most difficult two weeks of my life.

I slumped back in my bed in defeat.

"I'm so stupid," I said. "Why couldn't I tell you it was a…what was it?"

"A tripod."

"Yeah, a tripod."

"You're not stupid, Mimi," Kendra said. "This is a very common side effect with this kind of injury. The more we practice, the better you'll get at it."

This felt like a stronger pep talk than Tom Hanks would have given me in *A League of Their Own*. But I couldn't steel myself against feeling like a pathetic loser. In the past six months I'd lost my longtime boyfriend and my plans for a future with him, endured the intensity of graduation, and built up to a teaching career that had lasted about a week. Now here I was, screwing up a third-grade reading test. I wanted Spielberg or Howard or Scorsese to cut the scene and give me actor's notes. I wanted the expensive acting coaches to come in and revamp my character and portrayal of "Mimi Hayes, the courageous and inspiring teacher turned brain survivor."

It would have been easier that way, to pass the job to someone with a higher pay grade. But now it was just up to me. The therapists would push and encourage me the best they could during my stay here at Spalding. But in the end, it would have to be me.

## Robin the Bird

"Day two," I breathed into the camera of my Kindle. "I'm still in quarantine. There don't appear to be any survivors—" I heard a knock on the door and threw the Kindle under the covers.

"Here's your breakfast, Mimi!" the bright-faced kitchen lady said.

"Hey, thank you!" I smiled as if I wasn't just playing *The Blair Witch Project*. "What's your name?"

"Rosie!" Of course, it was; she was delightful.

"Thanks, Rosie!"

"Sure, Miss Mimi. Vicki will be here shortly to get you ready for PT."

The food was still tasteless on my tongue, but I ate it anyway because I figured I would need sustenance for another broomstick vaulting session. I'd decided after my first day in therapy to record some of my hospital antics with my Kindle. For one, it fueled my hopes that some Hollywood documentary filmmaker would pick it up and offer to take care of my student loans for good. I also wanted to *see* myself. Not in a narcissistic kind of way, but like a scientist sees her test tube samples under the microscope. I wanted to understand my body outside of my own comedic analysis. The only way to see what was going on with my brain was to catch it in the act.

"I haven't seen another real human in days. They're hiding something from me—"

"Mimi?" Vicki knocked and entered as I stashed the device again. "Let's get ready to go to the gym!"

My blockbuster documentary would have to wait. It was broomstick time.

Vicki handed me a new face mask, gloves, and smock to seal up my stank and keep it from infecting the other—and as far as I knew, nonexistent—patients.

We rolled into the gym and over to the exercise balls. At first glance, it was still a post-apocalyptic wasteland, but then I spotted an elderly man trotting behind a walker by the treadmills. I made friendly eye contact from underneath my bright yellow mask as we passed.

"Hello there, kiddo!" he said. I wasn't a fan of being the kiddo again, but it felt different this time with a cute old man saying it instead of Fake Phil, the world's worst physical therapist

I mustered a hi, feeling like a fungus in a petri dish.

"I'm Robin! You know, like the bird!"

"Hi, Robin the Bird. I'm Mimi." We exchanged smiles. Except you couldn't see mine because it was covered by the mask.

The results weren't back from the MRSA swab because someone hadn't had their coffee that morning and misplaced it. This meant a few more days in quarantine, my least favorite of all things. Robin the Bird was the first person I'd met besides my therapists and Rosie, the adorable kitchen lady. And I guess a few nurses who came by to stab me with needles every few hours. All right, I was surrounded by people. But it didn't feel that way. I was trapped and alone. Every time I looked out my hospital window, I remembered the life I wasn't living—playing in the newly red and orange leaves, walking Tucker, delivering life-shattering lessons to fourteen-year-olds. I used to be young and free, a happy-go-lucky character from a rom-com. Now I was just a germ trapped in a test tube.

Vicki helped me lock the wheelchair and instructed me to walk in a straight line on a strip of blue tape across the floor.

"You're walking pretty good there, kiddo!" Robin said from across the gym as he shuffled with his walker.

I peered over the exercise balls and wheelchair equipment at my new friend, feeling like a stranger in my own skin. What was I even doing here, all smocked up and stumbling over my own feet while an elderly man complimented me on my ability to take two steps without tumbling over? I couldn't imagine where my life would go from this and if I'd like my future at all.

I'd hardly slept the past few days, the brain steroids were so powerful; I'd spent months at home too, unable to sleep. Maybe my four-hour surgery would be the only rest I would get on my road to recovery. But the less sleep I got, the crosser I became. I'd only been here one day, and already I was sucking at physical therapy, crying in occupational, and feeling stupid in speech. I would have made an amazing actress—crying on command, laughing at inappropriate times, getting upset at the smallest of things. Every tiny victory and mountainous challenge brought with it a brand-new buffet of emotions. My range was fantastic. I could raise my hands in triumph at completing a single walking task and then start sobbing and thinking about how James left me and that I was a failure at life now. I needed a new friend to lift my spirits. So I fell in love with Robin the Bird, my very first old person companion.

Vicki told me to stay put while she ran to the printer to grab a new exercise. I didn't stay put. I unearthed myself from the unlocked wheelchair and onto a small blue bench several feet away. Robin and I continued to chat as he did tiny leg raises from his blue bench. Our conversation quickly ended when Vicki returned, her brow furrowed at my new "did not stay put" location.

"Meet me tomorrow," I whispered to Robin as she approached. "Dining hall. Seven o'clock." He winked, and I looked to Vicki with a not-so-innocent smile. Robin slunk away behind the exercise balls.

"What are you doing over here, Mimi?" Vicki asked as I squirmed on my blue bench.

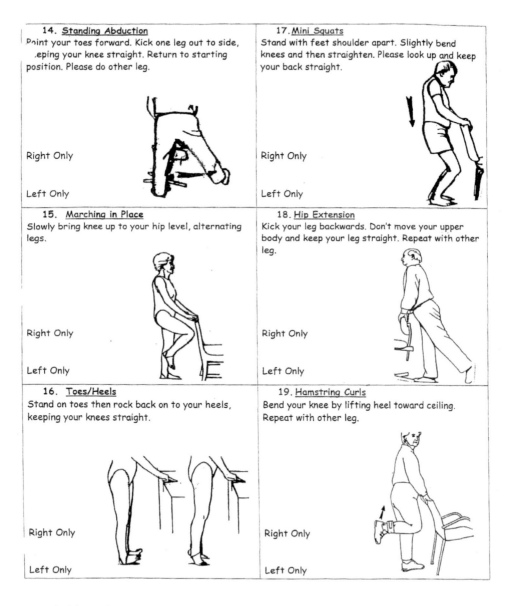

### 14. Standing Abduction
Point your toes forward. Kick one leg out to side, keeping your knee straight. Return to starting position. Please do other leg.

Right Only

Left Only

### 17. Mini Squats
Stand with feet shoulder apart. Slightly bend knees and then straighten. Please look up and keep your back straight.

Right Only

Left Only

### 15. Marching in Place
Slowly bring knee up to your hip level, alternating legs.

Right Only

Left Only

### 18. Hip Extension
Kick your leg backwards. Don't move your upper body and keep your leg straight. Repeat with other leg.

Right Only

Left Only

### 16. Toes/Heels
Stand on toes then rock back on to your heels, keeping your knees straight.

Right Only

Left Only

### 19. Hamstring Curls
Bend your knee by lifting heel toward ceiling. Repeat with other leg.

Right Only

Left Only

*Behold, my favorite physical therapy exercises with hand-drawn old people models.*
*Courtesy: Vicki Council.*

"I was making a new friend!" I said.

"Did you walk over to this bench by yourself?"

"Sure did!"

Vicki was not enthused by this small adventure. She told me I hadn't earned this kind of freedom yet and that I'd be in actual trouble if it continued. I apologized profusely, praying that my new friend was not nearby to see the spectacle.

Vicki helped me back into the wheelchair—after locking it—and then rolled me out of the gym. She assured me that she wasn't mad, just worried about my safety. I felt like a reckless idiot. The idea of meeting another patient had excited me so much that I'd ignored all rules and regulations. I'd forgotten that I wasn't supposed to do things like walk on my own. I was broken down and delusional. But I also wanted to do this right so that I could get myself out of this weird parallel universe.

I tried to shake off the ordeal and focused my efforts on the next day. I had a date with an old person! I was ecstatic. After Vicki rolled me back to my hospital room for my break, I took out a notepad and pen and prepped questions that I wanted to ask Robin, the wise and well-seasoned Bird:

1. World War II, were you there for it?
2. If you answered yes to question 1, where were you stationed? Did you ever fly a plane? Did you *kill a guy*?
3. Do you have grandkids? What are they up to these days? Do you have any cute male grandkids who are my age, by any chance?
4. What's your opinion on walkers with tennis balls on the ends?
5. Do you have an Instagram?
6. Do you know what #yolo means, and do you think it applies to your life?
7. What's your favorite film from the 1950s?

8. Do you remember what you were doing and wearing when Kennedy was shot?
9. Do you think you've aged well?
10. What were you like when you were my age?

I scribbled them madly on my notepad. I'd finally reached an age where old people were not just cute relics but rather a wealth of knowledge and wisdom that I could access. A fountain of untapped and elderly potential. Almost like a fountain of youth, but maybe the fountain had gotten a little rusty and occasionally spouted out brown stuff. Still works, right?

My MRSA swab finally came back clean, and I was allowed out of my test tube at long last. The stars were aligning in my favor; this would be my very first breakfast in the dining hall. *What am I going to wear?* I spread out my clothes on my bed and sat in my wheelchair looking at them. Running shorts, yoga pants, and baggy exercise shirts lay scattered before me. I had no need for jeans or tight-fitting clothing here in the hospital, not with my heavy sweating during the simplest of tasks. I certainly wasn't going to be attracting any fancy male suitors at Spalding. But I'd still be meeting Robin, and I didn't want to look like a fool.

I landed on a pair of black yoga pants to cover up my hairy legs and an old summer camp T-shirt. Then I rolled myself down the hallway to the dining hall. It was packed. I saw Robin down the line with his nurse in tow.

"Fancy meeting you here," I said, and darted behind him in line with a quick wheelchair maneuver.

"Hello there, Mimi!" He smiled.

Together we made our way down the line toward the food. It was my first time in this buffet line. I had PT with Vicki in thirty minutes, so I needed to stuff my face as fast as possible to get the most out of Robin's and my date. There was no time to get distracted by the—

"Salad! Look, Robin!" I yelled to him as we approached the start of the buffet. "They have salad!"

I made eye contact with Robin, my glasses tilting off my face.

Navigating the buffet line was harder than I'd thought. I didn't have a nurse pushing my wheelchair, so I had to focus on 1) wheeling the chair down the line without bumping into anyone, 2) reaching the food from my chair and placing it on my tray, and 3) figuring out what to do once I had all this food plus the heavy tray plus this stupid wheelchair. *Should I put the tray on my head and shimmy myself over to the table like a sexy waitress?*

A nurse standing at the end of the line must have seen the gears turning in my broken head. She offered to carry my tray to a table.

"Robin, where do you want to sit?" I asked as his nurse took his tray and began wheeling him away.

"Over here—this is my spot," he said.

I thought it was cool that Robin had a spot. *He must run this dining hall*, I thought. I reminded Robin to lock his wheelchair once we got settled.

"So you don't roll away," I said with a smile as I eyeballed my salad. It was ten after seven. Rehab made me a crave salad all the time, yet somehow I still managed to relapse into muffin top tendencies. Figured.

Robin and I sat together in that bustling dining hall and became best buds in approximately twenty minutes. I'd left the list of questions in my room, so I had to rely on memory. He told me about his family, his wife, and his grandson, who was a blossoming musician up in Boulder. He told me how he almost enlisted in World War II and would have deployed to Germany, when the war ended just in time. I did some quick and error-filled math in my head and deduced that he had to be lying about his age, or maybe he had forgotten how old he was. I figured I should go easy on him. He was probably just trying to impress me. Either that, or he had dementia. *Oh, Robin. You are adorable.*

We chatted between bites of bacon. I also learned that he grew up on a farm, loved to fish, and was an all-around delightful human being. He reminded me of Papa. I instantly relaxed. I stopped thinking I'd be trapped inside a hospital gym learning basic functions for eternity.

"When you bustin' out of this joint, kiddo?" he asked.

"Not sure," I said. "I guess it depends on when my brain heals. Maybe two weeks if I'm lucky."

"Two weeks ain't so bad, darlin'," he said. "I've been here almost two months."

"I bet you miss home. When are you leaving?"

"Tomorrow morning," he said.

My heart sank. "What? You can't leave me already, Robin the Bird! I just got here, and you are my only friend!"

Of course I was happy that Robin could go home. He had a wife and kids and grandkids who had been missing him for two months. But I was sad down to my core that my first and only hospital friend was leaving me so soon. It was a selfish feeling, to want an old man to stay in a hospital with me so that I wouldn't be alone. But my time with Robin had only just begun.

"Don't you worry about that, kid. You'll be outta here before you know it," he said, and smiled.

I sulked for the remainder of breakfast, slouching in my wheelchair and shoving my oatmeal around my bowl. We wrapped up our meals, and the nurses helped us clean up our trays. Robin and I rolled our way to the exit. This was it. The end of the line. Robin would be gone by the morning. But I had to do something, something big. Robin may have been ready to roll himself out of rehab, but I was ready for rebellion.

It had crossed my mind many times that I could break the sound barrier in my little wheelchair. While my legs were still dysfunctional, my arms were doing okay. I could text fine and was starting to type this book with more ease and coordination. My vision was still double, but they'd given me new tape to put over one side of my glasses so that my brain was tricked into seeing singular. Robin's nurse had left him to wheel himself back to his room alone, and the hallway was clear. This was our only shot.

"How fast do you think these puppies can go, Robby, ol' pal?" I said with a devilish glance toward the open stretch of hallway before of us. "You wanna race, Bird Man?"

He smiled back in quiet reverie, and we lined ourselves up in front of the nurse's station. I counted down in suspense.

"Ready?! Three…two…one…*gooooo!*"

We were off, our arms thrusting the wheels in a mad fury as we giggled down the corridor. I didn't even care if we got in trouble for this. Robin was busting out the next morning, and the nurses could do what they wanted with me.

When we reached the exit sign at the end of the hall, we called it a tie, laughing, and took a few deep breaths—we were both completely out of shape. I attempted a high five, although my double vision made it a bit off kilter and I skimmed his shoulder instead.

"Good run, my friend." I was breathing heavily.

Then came the time for our goodbyes. I've always hated this part. I can be a bit dramatic when it comes to saying goodbye to people. Apparently when I said it to my college friends in Minnesota before I transferred home to Colorado, I wrote them all speeches that I tearfully recited to each of them in the dorm lobby. I'd totally forgotten about that. What a sap.

"I'll miss you," I said.

"You'll be okay, kid."

Robin the Bird turned his wheelchair around, and I watched him as he rolled down the florescent-lit corridor and out of view. And just like that, my friend was gone.

That first morning out of quarantine taught me a lot. It taught me that someone could see me beneath the latex gloves and face masks. Robin saw me at a time when I desperately wanted to be invisible. I didn't want the life that I'd been living for the past two months. I didn't want intimate knowledge of how hospitals worked or how loud and scary the ICU could be. I wanted to fade quietly back into whatever confused and seemingly comfortable life I'd lived before. But Robin saw me anyway. He saw me, and he understood me.

Robin the Bird, Bird Man, Robby, keeper of my soul and first in my heart, if you are reading this, I hope you are out on a lake somewhere fishing like you said you wanted to. I hope your grandson is doing his music and making it big. I hope he's cute, and I hope you give him my number. I hope you live the rest of your days racing other fun old people in the aisles of grocery stores and making tons of friends. And most of all, I hope you know how much your kindness meant to me that day in the gym next to the exercise balls. Fly free, my friend. *Fly free.*

## The Poop Chapter

Everybody gets so uptight about fecal matter. Literally. People strain. I don't understand why everyone freaks out about poop. Our bodies can take food, partially digest it, convert it into energy, and dispose of the waste. Poop is our body's way of taking care of us. Poop is a beautiful thing. Can you imagine if all that yucky stuff stayed inside our tummies? We'd combust.

I'd never thought much about poop until I was incapable of doing it. For several days I'd been trying to relieve myself, with no success. The nurses explained that it was due to all the drugs I was on post-surgery. I felt, well, like shit. I was sure all the hospital food was stacking itself on top of my vital organs, ready to topple over.

By this point I'd become accustomed to discussing my bowel movements with strangers. When you're in the hospital, your business becomes everyone else's business. If you don't poop, you're not healthy, and if you're not healthy, you're certainly not getting a golden ticket out of this joint. I became fixated on the idea and even took it a step further. *If you don't poop, you're never living a normal life again.*

Nurses kept asking me about my bowels, and I kept disappointing them and myself. I was getting desperate. I was willing to try anything. Probiotics, stool softeners, poop pills, I did it all. I was committed.

"Has the miracle of life occurred yet?" Katrina chuckled over the phone on day six of the no-poo parade.

"Don't patronize me," I said. I was getting really sensitive about the shit situation. And the more I stressed about it, the less successful I became at summoning my inner demons. Shit's ironic.

Every time I felt a gurgling in my tummy, I'd move quickly—to my walker, not in my shorts—to the toilet. I would plop myself down on the bowl and try not to worry I'd be stuck in poo purgatory forever. *This is so great. I'm about to go number two.* I'd brace myself for impact, then…nothing. I wanted to curse the heavens. *Damn you, poop gods! Just let me be!* But I had to be patient. The nurses had told me not to strain myself. Straining is bad for your brain, apparently.

I waited eight long days before experiencing the reckoning. And when it came, I shouted from my seat at the glorious, shiny bowl. "Vicki, it's happening! It's coming out like a freight train!"

I must have spent forty-five minutes on that toilet, easily. Maybe even fifty. It was absolutely transcending.

Pooping became a form of meditation for me. I don't get why people are ashamed of it. Poop is the most miraculous thing in the world. It lets us know that our bodies are healthy and moving in the right direction. Is it a little yucky? Oh, sure. Nobody's shit smells like roses, not even Beyoncé's. But I bet it *does* smell like something powerful. Like strong coffee, maybe.

Losing the ability to experience this form of meditation taught me just how precious poop could be. It also taught me how badly constipated I had become in other ways. I'd been unable to poop for about a week, but hadn't I been emotionally constipated for five whole years? Was I just that unable to relax and let go? Maybe I'd been harboring relationship toxins for so long that I'd forgotten how to shit them out. And no amount of prune juice or awkward blind dates could change that. It's a grotesque image, and I'm not entirely sure my mother will appreciate this chapter, but it's important to note that this wasn't the first time I was bottling things up, intentionally or otherwise.

We know what's best for us in life and relationships—and in the bathroom. But we don't always know how to hunker down and get on with our business. We can't believe our dating/dinner choices led us here in the first place. We want a stable and loving significant other just like we want that damn beef taco to leave us in peace. This is getting very graphic, and again, Mom, I am *sorry*.

## Prune Juice, Saltines, and Ginger Ale

I don't have an entire chapter to write about these things. You should just know they are all items that they give you in the hospital to help you poop.

## Pissing Off Therapists

The large gym in the rehab center became my playground. I balanced on a moving platform. Vicki and I played Wii Sports. I even threw a ball across the room to her while I rode an electric bull. I thought the bull was a strange choice for a hospital, but I had a lot of fun riding it. In speech and occupational therapy, I slowly overcame my double vision and made brain logic puzzles my "female dog."

But it wasn't easy convincing my body of my limitations. Despite feeling like Rocky in an awesome training montage, I still lacked motor functions and general coordination. I didn't think through my movements; I simply moved, or tried to. I was getting better at it, but half the time I was still attached to Vicki with a gait belt like I was her camel.

Therapy was also more exhausting than I had bargained for. Because I'd never sat still in my pre-hemorrhage life, I rejected the idea of downtime now and found ways to occupy my day outside of therapy too. When I wasn't doing eye exercises with Jamie or playing Sudoku with Kendra, I was hobbling around my room watering my dying plants or binge-watching *How I Met Your Mother* or forgetting to lock my wheelchair correctly. Because who needed to lock a wheelchair when you had two fully dysfunctional legs not to get you places?

The locking of the wheelchair was a big to-do in rehab. As were a lot of rules that were created so that, you know, I wouldn't accidentally kill myself. But rules, as they say, are meant to be broken. I may not look like it now, but back in rehab I was the ultimate troublemaker. The reckless hooligan. I was a Hollywood starlet whose name I can't list here or I'll get sued, minus all the drugs. I mean, I was still on drugs. But they were a necessary coincidence to offset my swelling brain tissue.

Hospitals have some serious rules, it turns out. Rules about when you can go to the bathroom, rules about when you can eat, rules about when you can sleep and not sleep, rules about when you get stabbed with a needle. And they are all intended to keep you alive and well, even if you don't know what's good for you just yet.

But twenty-somethings don't believe in rules. We know they exist and everything, we just disregard them entirely. We know we should stop socially chain-smoking at rock concerts. We know we shouldn't text and drive. And yes, we even know to call on Mother's Day. But alas, our brains are still developing. And we'd rather not follow the rules now while we're still young and stupid.

I was quite counterculture in my adolescence and followed the rules thoroughly. Maybe I suffered from middle child syndrome and felt that any mistakes my older sister made, I had to atone for by being a dainty angel. But I liked being good, too. If a teacher ever called me out for chatting with a neighbor, I would sob and apologize for the rest of the school year. I didn't like feeling as though I'd hurt someone else. This is called uber-empathy disorder. Just kidding. I made that up. But I was seriously a good child. Naturally it came as quite a shock when I got to rehab and started giving nurses and therapists a run for their money.

It's not that I meant to be a sinner. My body just couldn't understand what my brain was going through. As a twenty-two-year-old, I took my ability to move gracefully for granted. I'd never had to put effort into sending brain waves to my body parts to move them. I'd never needed assistance doing anything or getting anywhere. I was self-sufficient. Or I had been.

I started out with minor infractions, like not asking for nursing assistance to readjust the ice pack on my neck. This resulted in the bag rupturing and sending freezing cold water all over my back and onto the bed. I also continued texting, even though I was advised not to expose myself to extraneous stimuli. This was almost impossible to resist, as hospitals provided the perfect backdrop for my hilarious

Snapchat series, "Late Night with Mimi: Road to Rehab."

It wasn't long before I tried breaking the biggest rule of all: DO not under any circumstances GET OUT OF BED WITHOUT NURSING ASSISTANCE. I repeat: do not DO IT. If you're reading those last two sentences from a distance, you can see how I got confused.

The thing about brain injuries is that you become a fall risk by doing just about anything. Moving, thinking about moving, thinking about thinking about moving; all put you at risk of slipping your way to a hilarious death. So you get a fancy yellow bracelet to let the world know that you are no good on your own. I still have mine. Two of them, actually. I wear them to parties sometimes and do my coordination exercises for my friends when I'm drunk.

I paid no mind to the "no walking without assistance" rule. I suppose I truly believed I could do just fine without working legs. I'd make slow, often painful attempts to get to the restroom on my own, only to find that the bed was equipped with motion sensors that beeped if I tried to leave it without help. I'd ignore them and move not so swiftly on with my journey to the toilet. Frequently I'd be intercepted by a worried and out-of-breath nurse at the door. Their expression would shift from worry to disgruntlement.

"What're you doing out of the bed, Miss Mimi?" they'd chide as I puttered aimlessly around the room, trying to find the bathroom.

"Just out for a stroll," I'd say. "Lovely day, isn't it, Nurse Person?"

~

My misdeeds continued unchecked for seven days, until I broke the biggest rule of all.

The process at Spalding was that you moved your way up through different modes of transportation. First was wheelchair with assistance. Next you removed the legs of the wheelchair; then came the walker and then the cane, and finally you graduated to a single-floor walking badge. Taking a walker to the dining hall when you were supposed to use a wheelchair was like giving a race car to a newborn. It just wasn't done. I mean, unless you're Bruce Willis's kids. Those children were probably drag racing by the time they were toddlers.

But I was getting another story in my head about what recovery was supposed to look like. One week's worth of scenes in a wheelchair was fine for a movie. But two? Nah. I was over it. So I threw caution to the wind.

It was quite an endeavor to get down the hall that morning. Not because anyone stopped me, but because I truly wasn't ready for the walker. My eyes still struggled to track objects in motion, and my gait was crooked and unstable. I moved slowly past the nurse's station, avoiding eye contact with anyone who might notice the unacceptableness of my taking the walker down to my egg and blue cheese salad morning ritual.

*What a beautiful tray you have this morning,* I said to myself as I moved carefully down the buffet line, acquiring all my favorite foods. As far as I was concerned, I'd carried out the perfect crime. Nobody had gotten shot in the getaway scene, and I could eat my meal guilt-free. I slid my tray toward the end. Rosie scanned my bracelet bar code and gave me a smile.

"Walker today!" she said.

"Oh yes!" I smiled to hide my mischief.

The greater challenge was holding the tray while pushing the walker once I left the buffet line. I'd neglected to consider this obstacle when I grabbed handfuls of butter squares for my rolls.

"Would you like help to your table?" Rosie asked.

"No, that's okay!" I smiled like the Cheshire Cat as I held the tray with both hands and attempted to push the walker toward the tables with my stomach.

By the time I reached the table, I was exhausted but proud. I hadn't dropped anything. I'd obviously shown that I had no limitations and that this whole brain hospital nonsense was just some weird psychological experiment set up by my psychologist mother to test my intelligence. She was probably hiding under the buffet table, taking notes on a clipboard during the whole ordeal.

"Five sticks of butter per roll," she'd jot down. "Very typical for someone with acute impulse control—"

"Mimi." Vicki's voice rang from behind me.

"Hi, Vicki," I said, focusing on unsticking the glorious golden wrapper from a pat of butter.

"Are you ready for physical therapy this morning?"

"Almost," I said. "I got a slow start, so I just need a few minutes to eat."

"Sure," she said. But I could hear the leveling of her tone. "Mimi?"

"Yeah, Vic?"

"How did you get here this morning?" she asked, her voice lowering an octave, like my mother's does when I do something really fucking stupid.

"I walked," I said, keeping my eyes locked on the butter, which was now slipping around my fingers.

"You walked." It wasn't a question. It felt as if she'd told me which friendly nurse I'd just beheaded before buttering my dinner roll.

"I did."

"And your wheelchair is—"

"In my room." I tried to hurry the words out of my mouth as if they would sting me if they stayed on my lips.

Vicki could have done a lot of things to me in that moment. She could have slapped me across the back of my stitched-up head. She could have yanked the chair from under me like cool guys do in movie scenes. But instead she knelt before me and grabbed my hands, forcing me to abandon my buttery distraction. Her gaze pierced through the tape on my glasses. I could feel her peering into the back of my bruised cerebellum.

"Mimi," she said. "Never, and I mean never, do that again."

"But I just—"

"Listen to me," she said. "Do you know why you can't do that?"

"Because it's not allowed." Tears welled up in my eyelids.

"No." She gripped my hands tighter. "Because you're in my hands now. And until you can do things on your own, it is up to me to keep you safe. I can't do that if you break the rules; do you understand?"

I nodded sheepishly. My butter cube had melted on the table, but I didn't care now. I felt pathetic and stupid. I hated being in a wheelchair, and worst of all, I hated that a week of rehab hadn't cured me. I wanted to be outside, breathing in the fresh autumn air, picking apples, or doing some other basic white girl fall shit.

I knew I was still being incredibly impatient with my body. I knew I had to stop hating it at every opportunity. Taking the walker out for a field trip before I was ready might have been harmless this time, but Vicki was right. One misstep could cost me my brain, and I was sure neither of my parents could afford to get me a new one this time.

## Youngbloodz 4 Life

Young people don't appreciate being young. Youthfulness is often seen as a disadvantage to us under-thirties. I correct bouncers at bars with vigilance.

"Of course I'm old enough to be in this bar. I'm twenty-three. I'm almost *too* old to be here, you peasant!"

Although youth can be correlated with immaturity, it also means you're awesome. I say this in terms of physical ability. I have been known to curse at small children on ski slopes as they zoom by with ease: "How dare you conquer this black diamond better than me! I go to the gym once a month, you little shit!" This is not something we appreciate while we are in the best shape of our lives, so it's no wonder that old guys get so uptight about kids frolicking on the lawns that took them hours to manicure in the scorching sun.

I've never been able to bound up and down mountains gracefully; anyone who has ever hiked with me knows this. And doing athletic tasks got even harder during my brain days. My hilarious hiking adventures were over. Even readjusting my pillow turned into an Olympic event. Things I'd never even had to think about before became the most mentally and physically exhausting chores I'd ever done.

"Walk up this ramp," Vicki ordered.

"Stand on this board."

"Hold your right leg in the air for five seconds."

"Get out of the wheelchair and walk to the table."

These were simple requests. Vicki wasn't asking me to run a half marathon or climb a mountain or strap on my old ice skates and stop some hockey pucks. I felt like a buffoon and a failure. To me, any progress that I was making in the therapy gym was overshadowed by the fact that I was there in the first place.

"I suck at this," I wailed at Vicki from atop a balancing board as she held me steady. It was my ninth day at Spalding. I'd thought surely I would have escaped through the ceiling tiles by then.

"You're doing better than you think, Mimi," she said.

"Wow, you're already doing the balancing board?" Karen called from across the gym as I teetered anxiously on the wooden platform.

Karen—my newest pal, a seventy-seven-year-old paralegal—was sweet, but I was getting frustrated. I knew it was ridiculous to ask the universe for a cute twenty-something brain-injured hockey player to come cross-checking into my wheelchair this afternoon, but I craved someone who understood my angst at being in an old folks' hospital at all.

I tried to shake off my loneliness and made my way to my wheelchair in the corner of the room. Maybe a salad with extra blue cheese would make me feel better, I thought. I wheeled myself down to the dining hall slowly, using my legs to scoot me along, since Vicki had removed the leg rests. It was no pass to freedom, but it was a big step forward.

I arrived to see the regular crew. Steven and Denise were by the TVs, the lady who talked in numbers was in the corner, and Rosie was delivering food trays up and down the halls like a saint. I grabbed my tray and went straight for the salad.

Suddenly I heard a voice—a young voice—coming from somewhere behind me. "Yeah, man, I like the food here, it's pretty good…"

"Tell us what you want and we'll grab it for you, dude," another young voice said.

I craned my neck and readjusted my glasses so that the piece of clear tape was directly on the lens over my right eye.

"Is that a youth I hear behind me?" I said as I struggled to rotate my wheelchair to where I could see his face while still keeping my tray balanced on my lap.

"Yeah. Youngblood right here," he said with pride.

"Hey, Youngblood. I'm Mimi," I said. "Do you mind if I sit with you today?"

"Of course, Youngblood!"

I liked that we had nicknames. It felt very hip.

His friends wheeled him over to a table and I joined them, eager to see a bit of life in this place. We began the standard first meeting exchange, a game I liked to call "How'd you end up here?" followed shortly by jailbreak plotting. The conversation began as you might expect:

"How'd you end up here?" he said.

"Killed a dude with a bendy straw," I said. "You?"

"What?!"

"Just kidding. I had a brain hemorrhage in my cerebellum."

We swapped juicy gossip on our favorite nurses, compared scars, and then moved on to the plotting part: when we expected to break out of the joint, or in other words, when they would let us leave.

I'd had similar conversations with a multitude of people during my stay at Spalding, and I'd fallen in love with every old person I met. It was amazing to speak with men and women who knew of a time before Siri, a time when you had to look people in the eye when you talked to them. But I was delighted to meet Youngblood that day.

His name was Alex. He was sixteen, and he'd been hit by a drunk driver while crossing the street. He'd suffered several brain hemorrhages and internal bleeding. His leg was broken in multiple places and had had to be reconstructed. They'd opened his skull too, to relieve pressure in his frontal lobe. Much of this he didn't remember. He couldn't recall how long he was in the intensive care unit. He didn't know what day he'd had surgery on his leg to insert metal pins and rods. He didn't remember the emergency airlift to the hospital in a helicopter or anything about the accident at all. Yet despite his lack of tangible knowledge, he was a beacon of lighthearted joy, joking with his friends about how he wanted to decorate the cast on his leg for prom season and occasionally trying to flirt with the young nurses. He never once held hatred for the person who'd nearly ended his life on the street that day.

I liked him immediately. His age put him in the ballpark of my students back at school. I pictured him causing a ruckus in my classroom and me smiling and letting him off the hook for not getting his homework in on time. He was like a little brother too, close enough in age to my own. I wondered what sports he played and if he was talking to any girls yet. I had the occasional urge to smack him in the back of the head for being immature.

Youngblood and I understood each other on a different level, connected in a way I couldn't with anyone else in the facility. Humans naturally expire. Shit falls apart. Until my children or my children's children discover the fountain of youth, we are all bound to become one with the earth. Having trouble walking, seeing, and forming logical sentences—I figured that when I got old, I'd grow accustomed to this kind of thing.

I wasn't supposed to be decomposing at twenty-two. I wasn't supposed to know about catheters or blood pressure cuffs or stool softeners. Alex wasn't supposed to get hit by a drunk driver at sixteen and be forced to relearn everything he once knew. Our youthful normal was turned upside down alongside our vision, and mine was still slowly trying to correct itself.

It seemed so wrong for us to be sitting in the dining hall of a neuro-hospital, chuckling about our lack of physical and mental function. He'd tell me how hard it was to learn to use a wheelchair, and I'd describe the time a nurse dumped an entire bag of IV fluid on me and then accused me of pissing myself. We decided that having a brain injury was the pits. It brought me peace to know that I wasn't alone, even though our recoveries, like our brains, were very different.

Alex wanted to go to prom without looking strange with his scars and the pins in his leg. I wanted to get back to my classroom and be student teacher of the year and not fear broomsticks and inanimate objects as tripping hazards. He was trying to ease back into a full school load by catching up on homework in the hospital, which left him overwhelmed and fatigued. I was trying to do lesson planning activities with Jamie and doubted that the crap I wrote down would make any sense to my students back home. We wanted to get back to normal, whatever that might be, as soon as possible. Youngblood and I were scared. We wondered what our lives would look like when we left Spalding and entered the unknown.

After that first meeting in the dining hall, Youngblood and I became hospital buddies. We were in different wings of the facility, so we mostly saw each other in the dining hall or in the gym during therapy. Our friendship existed in the moments we ran into each other around the hospital. It was a convenient friendship. A lot of our therapy schedules lined up, leaving us on opposite sides of the gym, chuckling at the other doing leg raises or practicing fifth-grade math equations. Or in my case, playing hide-and-go-seek for a TV remote with Vicki.

Attached to the gym was a small kitchen and a fake apartment designed to teach patients how to recover the life skills they'd need once they returned home. Here we practiced getting in and out of a shower properly, maneuvering around a kitchen without wrecking shit, and performing simple cooking tasks. I'd never considered the concept of life skills or that I needed to learn them. Everything I'd once done without thinking now had to be broken into simple and easily learned tasks. I was a two-year-old in a twenty-two-year-old's body with the stamina of a ninety-five-year-old. I liked the fake apartment, but it also scared me. It scared me to consider the possibility that I'd have to live with my parents for the rest of my life. Which honestly they'd quite enjoy. Soon enough they'd get old and fragile themselves, and I'd already be there to take care of them. Plus, we could take turns using the wheelchair.

See, there I go joking again. Really, it was a daunting thought.

I'd never have my own real apartment if I couldn't conquer the fake shower, makeshift kitchen, and '70s shag-style carpeted living room. I was sure Alex would struggle navigating all those damn complicated questions on the SATs.

"'Sup, Youngblood?" I puttered past him through the kitchen one afternoon, using my legs to move me in the chair as I mindlessly sent a text message with one eye open. We fist-bumped in a cute and uncoordinated way.

"Nothing much," he said, his face contorting. "Just trying to do this math problem."

I glanced at his paper and noticed a familiar set of numbers and symbols. Brain problems. As if we weren't bad enough at math and logic already, we were tasked with complex math scenarios that weren't even remotely relevant in the real world.

Let's be real. Nobody likes math. We don't even call it by its full name, mathematics. Because we're lazy and *math makes brain hurt*. And then your brain explodes and they force you to do *this* kind of shit:

## 9.

Four children (Ed, Marie, Natalie, Quentin) are different ages (9, 10, 11, 13), have different pets (cat, dog, gerbil, parakeet), and live in different kinds of houses (aluminum siding, brick, frame, stucco). From the clues below, see if you can find each child's name, age, pet, and kind of house.

1. Ed and the cat's owner play on the same team in Little League baseball.

2. Marie and the gerbil's owner live next door to each other.

3. The dog owner is two years older than the girl who lives in the house with aluminum siding.

4. The 11-year-old lives a block away from Quentin, who does not live in the frame house.

5. The parakeet owner's parents won't let her play football.

6. The brick house is two blocks from the 9-year-old's house.

7. Natalie, Marie, and the 11-year-old sometimes walk to school together.

8. The 10-year-old is a girl.

9. The cat owner is younger than the person who lives in the stucco house but is older than Marie.

©1978 MIDWEST PUBLICATIONS CO. INC.

## Chart for problem 9

|    | 9 | 10 | 11 | 13 | C | D | G | P | AS | B | F | S |
|----|---|----|----|----|---|---|---|---|----|----|----|----|
| E  | X | X | O | X | X | XO | ⦻X | X | X | X | ⦻O | ⦻X |
| M  | O | X | X | X | X | X | X | O | X | X | O | X |
| N  | X | O | X | X | ⦻O | X | X | X | O | X | X | X |
| Q  | X | X | X | O | ⦻X | ⦻O | X | X | X | O | X | X |
| C  | X | O | X | X | | | | | | | | |
| D  | X | X | X | O | | | | | | | | |
| G  | X | X | O | X | | | | | | | | |
| P  | O | X | X | X | | | | | | | | |
| AS | X | O | X | X | O | X | X | X | | | | |
| B  | X | X | X | O | X | O | X | X | | | | |
| F  | O | X | X | X | X | X | X | O | | | | |
| S  | X | X | O | X | X | X | O | X | | | | |

First of all, who even owns a parakeet anymore? Second, what on god's green earth is this? Alex looked up from his page and then back at me in dismay.

"I'm having a tough time with this, Youngblood," he said. "I never used to get frustrated at stuff like this." He set his pencil aside in defeat.

"I know, Youngblood," I said. "Just don't give up." We fist-bumped again, and I rolled over to Vicki in the fake living room to practice getting on and off couches.

"All right, Mimi," she said. "I want you to transition to the walker right here."

I locked my wheelchair and smiled to her. *See, I know what to do.* I grabbed the walker forcefully and hurled my body out of the chair.

"Boom!" I said, triumphant. But now I was dizzy. Vicki's face had multiplied by twenty-five, and I was in full-out tilt-a-whirl mode.

"Go back. Do it again," she said with wide eyes.

I was being reckless, of course. I still wanted to power through this stupid brain injury like a badass. Like Alex with his silly riddles, I wanted everything to go back to normal, and *now.* By the force of my own sheer will. I wanted the miniature Bruce Willis on my shoulder to light his cigarette and say, "Nice job, kid." This was not going to happen. I'd have to do it the un-Willis way.

So I started over. I unlocked and relocked my wheelchair, got a firm grasp on the walker, and shifted my weight carefully upward to a standing position. I even took extra time, moving the walker in steady increments rather than tossing it around the living room like I had before.

Youngblood chuckled from the fake kitchen table, and I darted threatening glances at him from behind my taped glasses. If it had been Robin, he'd have applauded my victorious walker maneuver. But Youngblood knew better. He knew this was ridiculous.

Vicki and I moved into the living room next. For twenty minutes we practiced sitting on the couch, getting off the couch, and moving from the floor to the couch and back again. It took forever. I was like a sloth after a bong hit. Muscles seemed to engage at DMV speed, post office speed, the speed at which teenagers look up from their phones and confront your existence. I focused on the brown suede stitches on the couch, then on the scruffy beige fibers of the carpet. I missed my own couch. I missed home and everything that had to do with it. I felt a pang of homesickness and despair as I crawled around the carpet. Was the rest of my life going to look like this? Taking twenty minutes to get on and off a couch in an old folks' home?

How could I possibly prepare for every single situation I'd encounter in real life? The transition from tile to carpet was a potential death zone. I was using a walker with tennis balls on the ends, for fuck's sake. I was an emotional basket case. I mean, I still am, but anyway, back to the carpet story.

Vicki sensed my frustration. "I won't be in your living room with you when you get home," she said. "You're going to need to do this the right way, or you could get hurt."

I knew she was right. Vicki wasn't always going to be there. And maybe that brought me a bit of ease, thinking of a day when I would no longer live at the hospital. If my functionality returned like they thought it would, I could go home in a week or so—could start my life again, even if with baby steps.

I thought back to my first day with Vicki, shuffling uncomfortably over broomsticks as she held me like a child trying to walk for the first time. I truly was a child. But my brain was healing every day, and with it my sense of confidence.

It hadn't occurred to me, but I'd made leaps and bounds since my arrival at Spalding just over a week before. Literally and figuratively. I'd gone from not being able to keep my head on my neck straight to walking in a line without falling over and even doing lunges with baby hand weights.

Youngblood proved to me the power of perseverance and laughter and pushed everyone around him to be better. He was my beacon, my fountain of youth, and my biggest inspiration, my friend when I was lonely, and my cheerleader when I thought I couldn't go on. Here we were, two young squirts feeling like old farts. We were the youngest kiddos in the establishment, and we understood each other, having both lost a bit of our youth in our injuries. It was the slowness of our joints, the confusion of moving into a room and forgetting why we were there. We tried to make the most of it together.

Later Youngblood accompanied me through outpatient therapy. We were in different programs and hardly saw each other, but whenever he appeared in the lounge, I was there with a smile and a sticker for my young groupie. I'd ask him about his return to school for half days. He'd ask if I'd found my Prince Charming yet. Of course Youngblood told me about going to prom, and how he'd decorated his cast and had all the pretty nurses sign it.

Eventually he left Spalding outpatient therapy and returned to school to finish the year, and I went back to my own classroom. I don't know where the little goober is today or what he's up to. I'm sad to say that I don't remember ever really saying goodbye. But wherever he is, I know he is loved well. *fist bump* *Youngblood outtttttttttttttttttt.*

## Brain 'Roids

I wrote pages upon pages of this book in my head long before I transferred them onto a screen. I wrote in beautiful prose; in vivid, grammatically correct sentences. It was really a lovely book, you see. I composed the whole thing in my swollen brain. And then I didn't write it down. I didn't write it down, because I was trying to sleep, not write a book. And as much as I liked the idea of a published book on a dusty shelf, I didn't want that shit going down in the middle of a REM cycle. I needed my beauty sleep.

I'd dabbled with insomnia in college, sometimes going two weeks without decent rest. It was more present with anxiety, though I could mostly manage it with Sleepytime tea, yoga, and over-the-counter sleeping pills. But I was perpetually grumpy at someone or something. Usually my roommates or the toaster. *The dang thing keeps burning my Toaster Strudel, and for the love of GOD, would you move your damn laundry out of the dryer already!*

Here at Spalding, it wasn't a final exam I was yawning through, but my eye exercises. And those kind of required my eyes to be open. My sleepiness was making me easily annoyed too, and the more tired I became, the shoddier job I'd do during physical therapy, frustrating me further.

My therapists even told me that my brain needed more rest than normal to heal from the injury. Then Nurse Lady Sunshine Bear would knock on my door at ten at night for the newest installment of sleep-depriving brain drug bullshit.

# Medication Chart

| Medication | For... | Dose | Schedule | Special Instructions |
|---|---|---|---|---|
| Acetaminophen (Tylenol) | Pain | As needed | → | Do not exceed 4 grams in 24 hours |
| Bisacodyl (Dulcolax) | Constipation | 10 mg (1) | As needed | Take if you don't go in 48 hours. |
| *? Maalox | GI Upset | 30 ml (1 cup) | As needed | '' |
| Magnesium Hydroxide | Constipation | 30 ml (1) | As needed | '' |
| Oxycodone/ Acetaminophen (Percocet) | Pain | 1 pill for Pain (3:25 3-6 mg) | As needed (every 4 hours) | Do not take more than 4 g in 24 hours. |
| Polyethylene Glycol (Miralax) | ? | 17 g | As needed | ? |
| Trazodone HCL (Desyrel) | Sleep | 50 mg (1) | At bedtime as needed | Do not take after midnight. |
| Calcium Carbonate (Tums) | Stomach | 500 mg (1) | As needed (twice daily) | ? |
| Cephalexin (Keflex) | Anti-biotic? | 250 mg (1) | ? | ? |
| Dexamethasone (Decadron) | Brain Swelling | 2 mg (4 pills) | Twice daily? *Just in AM | Take once in morning for — days |
| Docusate Sodium (Colace) | Stool Softener | 100 mg (1) | Twice daily | Take w/ plenty of water |
| Famotidine (Pepsid) | Gerd/ Prophylaxis | 20 mg (1) | Take at bedtime | |
| Heparin Sodium | Blood Thinner | 5000 mL (1) | Every 12 hours | *Can I get this in pill? |
| Lactobacillus Rhamnosus (Culturelle) | ? Pro-biotic | 1 cap | Twice daily | Cap may be mixed w/ cold drink or food. |
| Levothyroxine Sodium (Synthroid) | Thyroid | .112 mg (1) | Daily at 6am | *Wasn't I at .137 mg? ✓ |
| Medication | For... | Dose | Schedule | Special Instructions |
| Lidocaine/ Prilocaine | Numbing cream | Small dab | 4 times a day | Do not put directly on incision |
| Pantoprazole (Protonix) | Gerd/ Prophylaxis | 40 mg (1) | Daily at 6am | Do not crush pill. |
| Levora | Birth Control | (1) | Daily | |

*Who knew I'd find myself googling "Do I have GERD?" at two in the morning.*

At Spalding I had a lot of colorful pills to take: pills to help me poop, pills to numb the pain in the back of my head, pills to make sure my liver didn't shut off accidentally. I didn't understand what language the nurses were speaking when they rattled off the names of each pill as I swallowed them. Sometimes I thought about pretending to collapse dead after taking one of these mystery pills. My last words would be "Damn you, Nurse Teresa. Damn you to hell." But I never did. Vicki was already upset with me over the walker incident, and I didn't want to push my luck for a punchline.

Of all the pills on my long list, the steroids were the worst. They weren't new to me now; I'd been taking them at six, two, and ten every day since they'd found the damn thing growing in my brain like a demon space baby. Side effects? Not fucking sleeping.

Brain 'roids are no joke, you guys. This stuff is serious business. I'm talking wired awake, like Swiffer your entire house, clean out the pantry, vacuum your car, and build a mini Roman Empire out of waffles before sunrise. Sleep went out the window along with my sanity.

Sometimes when I couldn't sleep, I would try my hand at wheelchair tricks. I'd use my stumpy little legs to launch myself off the door and throw my hand inside the wheel to jolt it into a 180-degree spin. I was also recording myself on the tiny front-facing camera of my Kindle so I'd catch the glorious kick flip in action. Never you mind that one take when I wheeled myself directly into the trashcan. I meant to do that. Looked cool, didn't it?

After over a week of brain 'roids, my nerves were shot. The drugs kickstarted my neurons and made me want to run a goddamn marathon with my tennis ball–clad walker. I even wrote pounds of paragraphs in my head while trying to sleep on brain steroids. I did not make the wise decision to sit up and write anything down. That would have actually made sense.

Unfortunately some of my best work is gone completely, lost between raging brain waves in the dark abyss of my mind. Because I tried too hard to fight the system. I tried to beat the brain 'roids. It wasn't out of character for me to deny the obvious. No, you can't invent your own Prince Charming. No, you aren't Bruce Willis. And no, you can't force this drug to have no impact on your body. The drugs were there for a reason. They helped my brain balloon down to an acceptable size. I respected them. But that didn't mean I had to like them.

"Nurse Tiffany, my dear." I waved pathetically from the bed.

"Whatcha need, Mimi?"

"How much would you say these brain 'roids sell for on the"—I leaned forward—"black market?"

Okay, I didn't ask Nurse Tiffany that. I did ask if I could have some sleeping pills to counteract the brain 'roids like a druggy Sleepytime cocktail. Although I did the math in my head, and if I'd hoarded the 'roids under my pillow for long enough, I could have made a killing when I got out.

Sadly, the sleeping pills did little to soothe my constantly moving mind. Sleep became a rare commodity. I was miserable. My alarm in the mornings became more and more aggressive. I was moving so slowly during my rehab activities that I wondered if there was a secondary bleed or if I was just too fucking exhausted to function. Eventually I learned to sit up after several hours of not sleeping and jot down a note or a chapter heading for this book. But mostly I'd troll around Facebook and send a lot of hospital Snapchats and text messages at obscene hours. I figured I was doing my friends a big favor by showing them how interesting hospitals could be at three in the morning. Come on, you weren't sleeping anyway. You buncha jerks and your goddamn REM cycles.

I had a lot of time on my hands, time that I wasn't spending sleeping or writing.

You'd think I'd have invented a cool, hip gadget to rival the iPod or made that *Back to the Future* hoverboard. Maybe discovered a fun little bug in my toilet bowl. But no, I just spent hours talking to myself and balancing books (that I still haven't read) on my head to pass the time. Give me a break. I'm sure Bill Gates wasn't always solving the problems of the universe. And if he was, he definitely wasn't making a castle made of toothpicks at two in the morning. Because he was probably sleeping.

# The Chuckle of a Lifetime

*Wednesday, October 15, 7:01 a.m.*

The ticking of the clock resembled a hammer. My eyes were wide open. I'd been lying in the dark hospital room for hours now, trying to fight them closed. It was a lost cause. The breakfast line would soon begin; I had PT with Vicki a half hour after that. I accepted the fact that sleep was not happening for the duration of the day.

As I groped around in the darkness for stretchy pants and a clean shirt, my phone beeped, alerting me that I had a text message. I assumed it was from one of my friends, or possibly my mother was telling me not to trip on any weird rocks in the hospital garden today. I grabbed my phone off the charger and looked down at the bright screen.

It read "Text message from James."

To be more accurate, it read "Text message from Shithead."

I let out a tiny laugh and set my phone down on the bed. I put my glasses on in case my eyes were acting up again and I'd misread the screen. My eyes were always worse in the morning. It was entirely possible I needed to readjust the tape on my glasses over my right pupil.

I slowly picked up my phone and took a deep breath. Then I swiped the screen and clicked the tiny mailbox forcefully. I couldn't imagine what in the hell James would want to say to me now, of all the times in the world. Now, before my eight o'clock salad and my eight thirty walk with Vicki in the garden. I hadn't heard from him since he'd placed my sad belongings on my porch some four months ago.

By Wednesday, October 15, 7:01 a.m., I most certainly did not care for James being in my life. The breakup had left me in pieces, pieces that I was still haphazardly trying to put back together when my brain exploded. I didn't know what he'd say if he knew I still cried at night thinking about how much he'd hurt me, and that now my hurt was even greater. I didn't know what it would mean to him that I'd recently earned a second-floor walking badge and that Vicki had approved me from wheelchair to walker. I didn't know anything about him, and he didn't know anything about me either.

Maybe if I closed my eyes tightly enough, the text wouldn't exist at all. I shut my eyes for five seconds and then reopened them. Nope. Shit. Still here.

I sat up on the edge of the bed and read the text.

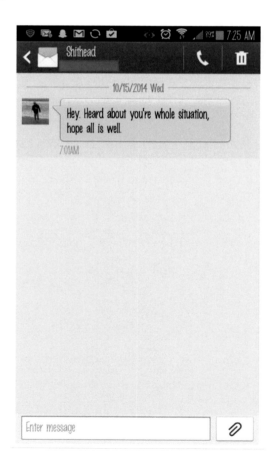

Before I continue, I would like to point out that there is a rule about these things. You're not supposed to respond. Because responding means that you still care for this person, which by now you obviously shouldn't. And nothing good can possibly come from texting with a sleep deficiency and one working eye.

By this point I'd received well-wishes, flowers, cards, visits, phone calls, text messages, grilled meats, Facebook chats, and more from just about everyone I knew. The love and support had been almost overwhelming. People I'd worked with at a coffee shop years ago were contacting me and wishing for my health and well-being. James's grandfather had come to visit me in rehab and given me a plant called a pregnant flea. All of James's work pals had sent me flowers, candy, and balloons and had come to see me throughout my recovery. I had a box of fucking grilled meats awaiting me at home from a group of complete strangers.

"Have you heard from James?" my friend Brittney asked the day after my surgery.

"No," I said coldly. "And you damn well know I would have been there if this were him." I flicked my finger at the yellow smiley face balloon she had tied to the foot of my hospital bed.

Of course, I sounded ridiculous. The idea that I'd want James showing up in my hospital room to hold my weak hands was absurd. I didn't want him around any more than I wanted Hugh Grant to come bursting through my door with his latest jerky monologue. I'm sorry. I hate that guy. He's not charming. He's just British. They are not the same thing.

In my mind I'd painted James into a beautiful Prince Charming masterpiece. But it was deceptive, and it always had been. He was neither the hero nor the villain. And I'd never be the hero of my own story if I couldn't snap out of my delusions.

When I looked down at the text message that morning, I laughed. I laughed and laughed and laughed. My lungs filled with air, and I filled them up again for more. I laughed for about twenty minutes. I laughed because what I really wanted to do was cry. I wanted to cry because he hadn't been there for me through all this. I wanted to cry because I suddenly felt deceived and alone. It didn't matter that I had Facebook friends asking about me or grilled meats in the freezer. James hadn't been here for me. He never would be. And if he tried, he'd be shot on sight—we all knew that. His small words on the screen seemed so dismal compared with the gaping hole he'd left in my heart just months before.

The truth was that the breakup had come at a convenient time, even if I didn't feel it on the night he smushed my heart. I'd never have left James of my own free will. I was too messed up. I'd spent years imagining him into exactly how I wanted him to be. And every time he'd shown me that he was not my muse, I'd grab my color palette and cake on more and more paint until the canvas oozed with lies.

If James had stuck with me through August, we'd have been truly fucked. My sickness would have guilted him into staying to take care of me; if he'd walked out then, he really would have been the villain. Then once I recovered, I would have believed that he'd been the one who'd gotten me through it. Then he'd leave. And I'd be pissed as hell, because he was supposed to be the hero, not the villain, and I couldn't possibly carry on in this new, unfamiliar world without my Prince Charming. *Damn you, fairy-tale brain!*

It was fate that James had made an exit before shit really went south. I'd had to go through it without him, and my stay at Spalding had proved to me that I could do just that. Jamie was right all along. I was brave.

But that didn't change the fact that I was still scared out of my puffy mind to be alone. I laughed at the text because part of my brain lit up and alerted me that I was sad, so it needed to expel a different chemical so I wouldn't burst into flames.

But then I stopped laughing. And I got angry. Angry that James would dare text me now, after all this. After the exchange of shit. After the new girlfriend flying in my face like a pesky Confederate flag. After I'd given up Berlitz and gotten him back in my shame. After a hot doctor had tooled around in my brain. Did James not know that distance was the only cure? That he'd 'have to avoid me like a prison sentence for me to ever be able to heal from this heartbreak?

I took another deep breath and began typing. I punched my thumbs onto the screen as slowly and deliberately as if he could feel the hatred with each letter.

"You're hilarious," I wrote, to make sure he could see his grammatical error. "Fuck off."

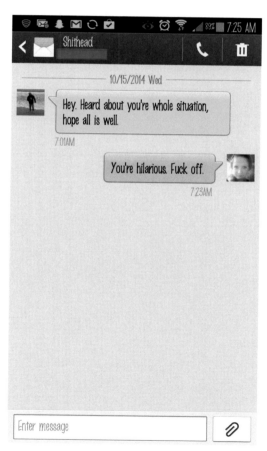

I hit Send and then rolled back in bed to resume my laughter. I threw on a shirt and wheeled down to the dining hall alone for breakfast, still steaming with crazed amusement.

"Good morning, Mimi," Vicki said as I shifted eggs aggressively from one side of my tray to the other. "How are you doing?"

"I'm doing fantastic." I grinned and threw my fork in the air. "Look who decided to join the party." I thrust my bright phone screen in front of her nose.

She took a step back, almost as if she was trying to decide where to put her feet next.

"Wow. This is"—she set her clipboard down—"really messed up, Mimi."

It was messed up indeed. It was messed up that despite everything—my delusional fairy-tale mindset that could never be real, the heartbreak that I'd had coming all this time, the head trauma that had left me useless and disabled—despite all these hurtful realities, I was still laughing.

## Your Chariot Awaits

A lot of bizarre shit goes down in the scene between Cinderella and her fairy godmother before the grand ball. Aside from the dancing pumpkins, mice turned into horses, and sing-songy incantations, Fairy Godmother is kind of oblivious. After changing literally every aspect of Cinderella's situation, Godmommy is somehow blind to the fact that Cindy herself looks like a ragamuffin.

Cinderella keeps trying to politely allude to the fact that all this stuff wasn't really what she meant by *transformation*. Her godmother even changes the dog before she looks to Cinderella. *This is bullshit, where's my dress, Godma?* Finally Fairy G realizes that raggedy Cindy needs some polishing up too and spins her magic wand, transforming her into the beautiful fake princess that she always wanted to be. Cinderella looks beautiful; her hair is all done up, and her dress twinkles in the moonlight. But alas, there's a catch. She's got until midnight. When the clock strikes twelve, it's over.

It is clever of the storyteller to bring an element of cruel reality to our otherwise fantastical fairy tale. Cinderella could have her night on the town, but she'd still be a housemaid at midnight. She could wear the glass slippers for the evening, but they weren't hers to keep.

I felt a lot like Cinderella on my last day at Spalding. Vicki and my therapy team had transformed a lot of things about me. They'd helped me upgrade from wheelchair to walker to cane. They'd cut the tape on my glasses into smaller and smaller pieces as my eyes grew adjusted to singular vision. My family and friends had helped me to transform as well. I was gaining the weight back, thanks to their cheeseburger delivery services, and I had a new collection of stuffed animals and potted plants.

Mom had even bought me new running shoes. They weren't glass slippers, and I wasn't allowed to run with them until December, but to me they were the most beautiful ballroom shoes of all.

But two weeks in intensive therapy had changed me more than I could comprehend.

"All right, this is the step test," Vicki said into my camera. "This is what Mimi looked like the first time she did the test."

On her cue, I pretended to stumble around the broomsticks, making sure to look like a fool. After knocking them about the floor, I carefully placed them back into position.

"Note how she can bend over," Vicki said. "She would have been on her face."

I repositioned myself at the start as Vicki prepared to time me for my final run. It had been two weeks since I'd done the broomstick test. My mind flashed back to how pitiful and ashamed I'd felt tripping over the sticks with Vicki that day. Part of me was still just as scared as I'd been before. These broomsticks represented everything in my life that I felt I couldn't overcome: my heartbreak with James, my failing body, and my uncertainty about my future as a functioning member of society. Vicki may have helped me heal my body, but she couldn't wave a magic wand and make those sticks go away. What I couldn't navigate was imagining what life would look like once I left this place. It felt like Everest itself.

"Here she goes," Vicki said. "The first time she did this test, it was fifty-two seconds. Eight seconds is the norm. Are you ready?"

"Ready," I said, and bent my knees in preparation.

"Ready, set, go!" She pressed the timer and held the camera up, and I leaped over the first stick, pressing my knees together at each turn and hopping from space to space like a glorious and graceful bird. I cut through the pattern as fast as I could while maintaining proper form. Vicki was always a stickler for proper form.

"Time!" she called as I stomped over the last stick and planted my feet squarely.

I was panting, shaking with excitement. If I'd beaten the broomsticks, I'd beaten everything. I could go home. Had my time been thirty seconds? Twenty-five?

"The step test that took you fifty-two seconds to do two weeks ago…"

"Yes…"

"Today you did the same test…"

"*Vicki, what's my time?*"

"Your time was 5.8 seconds!"

I let out a shout of victory. *5.8 seconds?* In just 5.8 seconds I'd tackled the thing that had made me most afraid. I felt like she'd just given me a golden tiara and sparkling hospital gown. It was the biggest success I'd ever experienced. I'd not only beaten my time, I'd crushed the normal time for non-brain-injured people. I high-fived Vicki with my more coordinated hand and danced around the gym like a happy fool.

My win over the broomsticks carried me into the rest of the day. I packed my gym shorts, stained T-shirts, and granny panties into my duffel with a smile and threw out the rotting flowers by the window. I looked to the wall, uncertain about taking down the corkboard of get-well-soon cards from my students of five days. A few months ago I'd envisioned my life in that classroom. A lot had changed since then. Would they rejoice at my return? Would they even remember me?

I resolved to write love letters to every single person I'd met at Spalding. Nurses, therapists, Rosie, Guy Who Drew My Blood One Time; they'd all get a farewell address. I still had a whole bag full of pumpkin chocolate chip cookies that I'd baked with Jamie a few days earlier in the fake kitchen. I'd leave them for the nurses and therapists as a token of my undying love.

# Pumpkin Chocolate Chip Cookies

## Ingredients

- 1/2 cup (1 stick or 115 grams) unsalted butter
- 1/4 cup (50 grams) light or dark brown sugar
- 1/2 cup (100 grams) granulated sugar
- 1 teaspoon vanilla extract
- 6 Tablespoons (86 grams) pumpkin puree (use the rest of the can in *any of these recipes*)
- 1 and 1/2 cups (190 grams) all-purpose flour
- 1/4 teaspoon salt
- 1/4 teaspoon baking powder
- 1/4 teaspoon baking soda
- 1 and 1/2 teaspoons ground cinnamon
- 1/4 teaspoon ground nutmeg*
- 1/4 teaspoon ground cloves*
- 1/4 teaspoon allspice*
- 1/2 cup (90 grams) semi-sweet chocolate chips

## Directions:

In a medium bowl, whisk the melted butter, brown sugar, and granulated sugar together until no brown sugar lumps remain. Whisk in the vanilla and pumpkin until smooth. Set aside.

In a large bowl, toss together the flour, salt, baking powder, baking soda, cinnamon, nutmeg, allspice, and cloves. Pour the wet ingredients into the dry ingredients and mix together with a large spoon or rubber spatula. The dough will be very soft. Fold in 1/2 cup semi-sweet chocolate chips. They may not stick to the dough because of the melted butter, but do your best to have them evenly dispersed among the dough. Cover the dough and chill for 30 minutes, or up to 3 days. Chilling is mandatory.

Take the dough out of the refrigerator. Preheat the oven to 350F degrees. Line two large baking sheets with parchment paper or silicone baking mats.

Roll the dough into balls, about 1.5 Tablespoons of dough each. Slightly flatten the dough balls because the cookies will only slightly spread in the oven. Bake the cookies for 8-10 minutes. The cookies will look very soft and underbaked. Keeping them in the oven for longer may dry them out. Remove from the oven and press a few more chocolate chips onto the tops, if desired. If you find that your cookies didn't spread much at all, flatten them out when you take them out of the oven.

Allow the cookies to cool for at least 10 minutes on the cookie sheets before transferring to a wire rack. The longer the cookies cool, the chewier they will be. I let them sit out for at least 1 hour before enjoying. I find that their chewiness and pumpkin flavor is more prominent on day 2. Cookies stay soft, moist, and chewy stored at room temperature for up to 1 week.

**Freezing directions:** Roll the chilled dough into balls and freeze in a large ziplock bag for up to 2 months. Baked cookies may also be frozen up to 2 months.

"Dear Vicki," I wrote. "How can I possibly write into words what you have done for me and my family these past few weeks…"

A few weeks. The first time Vicki and I met, I couldn't even lift my head out of the bed and was so tripped out that I called her Deana, an event we'd soon realize meant that we were fated to be together.

I looked to the rip-away calendar on the wall, which informed me that these champions had helped me completely transform my body and mind in just two weeks' time. It was October 16. I would have been turning in my teacher portfolio today. I would have been running a half marathon the following weekend. But I was going home.

In order for Vicki and the crew to send me on my way, we needed to run some final tests: eye exams, strength tests on the balancing board, and a final walk-through of the fake apartment. But the one I hadn't anticipated was showering with Marge. It sounds strange when I say it like that, but it's not what you think.

I had to pass a shower test to prove I could handle myself in the most dangerous place in my home: the slippery deathtrap tub/shower combo. This involved allowing a random nurse to watch me shower. I'd never been watched in such a vulnerable place before. Washing the disappointment of the day off my body was something I normally enjoyed in private.

A nurse I'd only seen in passing was the chosen one. I guess I was grateful that she wasn't one of my regulars, who would probably have had a good laugh at my hairy legs and gross athletic toenails.

"Do you mind if I shave my legs in here?" I asked, and inched the shower chair closer to the stream of water. "You don't have to, like, be anywhere, do you? Do you have kids?"

It turned out Marge was a nice lady in her late sixties. We exchanged banana bread recipes and had a lovely chat while I scrubbed my gooey little body, making sure to give the back of my head extra attention. The stitches had all healed now, but it was itchy back there. I had to be careful not to itch too hard, or I'd bust the seams and my brain would ooze out the back. I knew that wasn't how it actually worked, but I still feared that an alien was lying in wait behind the stitch marks, just holding on for the ideal opportunity to crawl its way out and roam the hospital, looking for a less brain-damaged host.

After my shower, the nurse checked a box on my discharge form.

Next was an explanation of my post-care medications and instructions. I felt like I was about to take a new baby home, except the baby was me.

"Make sure that you always have a friend or family member around when you're moving somewhere, so that they can assist you." Jamie read on from an extensive list, and I was pretty sure by the end of it that she was just looking around the room and pointing out all the things that might kill me.

"Sex," she said. I let out a small giggle.

"If you plan on being sexually active at any point in the future, make sure that your partner is aware of your injury and that you don't take things too fast and that you stop if you don't feel well."

I could just picture it now. Me and some unidentified male suitor parking a walker beside the bed. "Before we do this," I'd say, moving slowly onto the bed, "I'm going to need you to know that my head exploded a few months ago. It could happen again at any time."

"Are you sure about this?" he'd ask, because he'd be a respectable man who knew consent was sexy. "We don't have to do this if you aren't ready."

"Oh no, I'm ready," I'd say. "My safe word is *cerebral cortex*."

~

# SPALDING REHABILITATION HOSPITAL
## 900 POTOMAC ST.
## AURORA, CO 80011

### FINE MOTOR TAKE HOME SHEETS

### FINE MOTOR ACTIVITIES FOR THE HAND

The following activities are recommended to improve hand strength and dexterity. Look through the lists and select activities which interest you. Your therapist will check the ones which will iprovide the best exercise for you.

_____ Crewel/Embroidery
_____ Needlepoint
_____ Sewing by hand
_____ Cross Stitch
_____ Crocheting
_____ Knitting
_____ String Art
_____ Leather Lacing
_____ Macrame
_____ Jewelry Making
_____ Bead Stringing
_____ Turkish Rug Knotting
_____ Fly Tying
_____ Latch Rug Hooking
_____ Charcoal Drawings/Pastels
_____ Paint by Number
_____ Ceramic Painting
_____ Making paper mobiles/paper airplanes
_____ Tissue Paper Flowers
_____ Making yarn pompoms
_____ Putting together model kits
_____ Paper quilling
_____ Seed mosaic pictures
_____ Mosaic tile trays/trivets
_____ Making cloth napkins
_____ Woodworking projects using hand tools
_____ Card games
_____ Cribbage
_____ Making a card house
_____ Dominos
_____ Checkers
_____ Scrabble
_____ Chinese Checkers
_____ Backgammon
_____ Jigsaw puzzles
_____ Dial the phone, call a friend
_____ Type on an electric/standard typewriter
_____ Carry book between thumb & fingers

_____ Playing jacks
_____ Cat's cradle
_____ Etch-a-Sketch
_____ Lacing Cards
_____ Play dough
_____ Computer Games
_____ Sort buttons, sewing supplies
_____ Sort nuts, bolts, nails, etc.
_____ Peel potatoes/oranges
_____ Snap Beans
_____ Shell Peanuts, shrimp
_____ Cut Coupons out of paper
_____ Glue savings stamps in books
_____ Re-file recipe cards
_____ Polish silverware
_____ Use a manual can opener
_____ Re-pot plants and remove dead leaves
_____ Pick flowers or vegetables from garden
_____ Make bows for gifts
_____ Write letters, write in a daily log, make shopping list, record daily events
_____ Copy a favorite poem, recipe or story
_____ Trace a favorite design or picture
_____ Page through a book
_____ Tying knots
_____ Put photos in an album
_____ Put on make up, paint fingernails
_____ Eat popcorn — one kernel at a time
_____ Floss your teeth
_____ Replace shoelaces
_____ Roll your hair in pin curls or rollers
_____ Put keys on a key chain
_____ Turn off lights, turn door knob
_____ Open mail
_____ Peg games (Mastermind)
_____ Connect-the-dot games
_____ Use a calculator
_____ Do simple finger exercises on a piano
_____ Picking up coins of assorted sizes
_____ Turning screws

**SPALDING REHABILITATION HOSPITAL**

## Fine Motor Control – Home Program

1. Active range of motion: Extend fingers/thumb all the way and then make a fist. Spread fingers apart and then bring them back together.
2. Isolated finger flexion/extension: Place hand on table and lift each finger off the table (one at a time).
3. Opposition: Touch thumb to each finger (one at a time); gradually speed up to increase the difficulty of the activity.
4. Walk fingers up the wall or along countertop.
5. Writing/tracing: Write a letter or card to a friend or trace pictures/objects/letters of different shapes and sizes.
6. Lay coins on a table and then pick them up from the flat surface. Start by picking up one coin at a time, and as this skill improves, hold the coins in the same hand that is picking up the rest of the coins.
7. Piano scales: Push piano keys down and then lift finger off key. Begin with thumb and then index finger, then middle finger, and so on. Come back up the keyboard this time beginning with the little finger.
8. Play with cookie or pie crust dough. Roll it into a ball, stretch it out, pinch it, twist it, etc.
9. Type on computer keyboard or typewriter.
10. Make pinch pots out of clay.
11. Scissors activity: Cut out shapes, objects, pictures, etc. If you enjoy making scrapbooks, this is a great activity to improve fine motor control by: cutting, stamping, peeling stickers from one surface/placing on another, writing, tracing, coloring, etc.
12. Origami or paper airplanes.
13. Buttoning (buttons of different sizes), zipping jackets, lacing, and tying shoelaces.

## GAMES:

14. Card Games: Holding cards, sorting, and shuffling cards.
15. Chinese checkers
16. Operation
17. Board games such as Life or Monopoly where there are small pieces to handle helps work on fine prehesion and grasp.
18. Jacks

My last order of business was saying goodbye. I can't do goodbyes. Even now I don't think I've fully left Spalding Rehabilitation Center, because I keep showing up again. And saying goodbye. And then coming back. They just can't seem to get rid of me.

But for now I was all packed and ready to go; the only thing I needed to do was walk myself out the automatic doors. Despite my renewed walking abilities and slowly aligning visual fields, this felt an impossible task. Spalding represented so much more to me than a hospital; it was my saving grace. This place and these people had rallied behind me as I spent two weeks relearning how to do everything that used to be second nature. I missed home, but what would become of me if I truly went home? After everything I'd been through, how was I to leave this place?

The last time I'd been home, I was slugging around the living room, watching TV and spiraling into depression. Life had gotten real lifey since I'd left. I'd been through hellish MRI machines and back out. I'd learned how to tie my shoes again like a big girl, and I'd met some unlikely friends. Now I felt like I was leaving on a harrowing journey, and I was. I may have been going home, but the home I knew would look new and strange to me.

"Mom, turn the camera around," I said as my mother took accidental footage of her confused face with my phone. "Over here, get us hugging and me moonwalking to the car."

A nurse helped me pack my belongings into the Tahoe, and Mom videoed me dancing out the double doors and into the parking lot.

"Well," Mom said as we rolled away from my temporary home. "Are you ready?"

"Yes," I said. "Ready as I'll ever be."

## Squeaky Clean

"Sweetheart," Mom called to Dad from the garage. "Get the dogs; I don't want them knocking her over when she comes in."

"Move slow, baby," Mom said to me as she opened the car door.

I hadn't been home in just over two weeks. It might as well have been two years. I'd never wanted anything more than to be back in that house again, yet I was terrified to cross the threshold now.

I walked deliberately, like a tightrope walker, to the door, my heart galloping in my chest. Mom opened the door gingerly, and then I felt the warm, low light of the laundry room hit me like a familiar high five. The quiet of it all put me at ease. There were no beeping beds or strangers climbing the walls. I'd never realized how much I fucking loved that about this place.

Once I was seated in the kitchen, my family around me, Tucker and Erin's dog Leelou rushed over to assess my condition. Tucker was more relaxed than he'd been during his hospital visit the week prior. This calmed my nerves, because I understood now what I hadn't before: that he'd been worried about me. Today he was excited to see me. He sniffed my stained clothes and licked my hand.

There was a new sense of freedom here that hadn't been present at Spalding. I'd been emancipated from the chains of florescent lights, needles, and stiff sheets. I'd left behind the pressure cuffs and fall risk bracelets. Nothing could hurt me here. No one would make me walk on a treadmill or get up early to take brain pills. I still had to do these things. But now I could do them on my own terms.

The first thing I wanted was a shower all by myself. But this was a risk. The last time

I'd showered was with *Marge*, and I wasn't about to go back to Spalding to ask for more stories about her children while I washed the hospital stank off me. All other showering had been done under the watchful eye of nursing staff in bathrooms with shower chairs, rooms with panic buttons hanging above the toilet. I'd always had someone to hand me the soap and help me wrap my hair in a towel. And even though I'd practiced getting in and out of a shower solo in the miniature apartment during PT, I'd been working with props. There'd been no running water or soap-in-the-eye scenarios.

"Can I take a shower?" I asked my parents when the dogs calmed down. "It's all I want in the world right now."

"I don't want you using your shower upstairs yet," Mom said. "Why don't you use the shower in Dad's office?"

I entered Dad's office and moseyed past his rolls of architect designs and drawings. Just a few years ago he'd finished this attachment to the house, originally meant for my grandmother when she was living with us after Papa died. My father fully furnished the space, and it became her own little apartment with a bathroom, shower, the whole works. For a time, Grammy's apartment seemed to be working out, but she was so miserable after losing Papa that she would barely come out of her room.

Grammy began to get sicker, falling and breaking her hip, which ultimately led us to move her to an assisted living center—which I would soon discover was *not* the same thing as a brain rehab center.

"It's a walk-in, so you won't trip in the tub," Dad added. "You can even sit on that little ledge and use the shower hose."

Hoses and chairs had once seemed excessive to have in the shower, but I welcomed the offer now. It was better than having my mother scrub my armpits. I knew she'd do it if I asked, but I'd already traumatized her enough with my hair falling out in the first post-surgery shower.

"Here," Mom said, handing me a box. "From my friend Susie." I opened the box to find a fuzzy cheetah-print robe. Now I was extra excited for this shower.

"Dinner will be ready once you're done," Dad called before I turned on the water. Of course it would be. My dad was a goddamn champion.

I hung up my robe and stepped carefully inside the shower, and as the water touched my skin, I let out a sigh of relief. The hot water felt like a rebirth. It was the most fabulous sensation I'd known in months. Better than the PT successes and friend visits and gifts. I was clean. I could wash the hospital smell off me, hopefully for the last time. I sat on the little ledge, clutched the hose between my knees, and let the water cascade over my legs as I scrubbed shampoo into my head. Every bitter memory of pain and suffering seemed to slide off me and swirl around the shower drain. For the first time in a long time, I wasn't dizzy. I was just still. Present in the moment and completely centered.

That shower must have lasted at least forty minutes. It was so wonderful, I didn't want to leave. But at last I carefully wrapped a towel around my head and swaddled myself in the fuzzy robe. When I waltzed through the kitchen, feeling like a pampered goddess, my mother looked at me like I'd just come home from war. In her mind, a forty-minute shower surely meant that I'd slipped on a bar of soap and impaled myself with the shower hose.

"You do okay in there?" Brian asked.

"Oh, I did more than okay," I said. "I did fantastic. I feel like a new human."

## Heating Pads and Handrails

When you get hurt, your friends and family make valiant attempts to heal you, or at least make you comfortable. They try not to laugh when you find yourself incapable of giving high fives. They're not doctors, so they can't mend your broken parts. But they can readjust your ice baggy and bring you cheeseburgers that you immediate inhale because your appetite is back and with a vengeance.

The day I got home, my dad went into superhuman mode again. Anything I needed, he did without question. I asked for a yogurt once, and he stocked the fridge with twelve. Dad spent an entire Saturday installing handrails and a shower chair in the office shower like it was no big deal. My dad is the *man*. And he does this without thinking, because he's the best person I know.

I have been extremely lucky to have people in my life who've given me what I needed when I needed it. But it's bigger than that. These people didn't get anything out of running my errands. Nobody told them to. It wasn't a chore. They did these things because they loved me. That's the definition of unconditional love.

Back in college my roommates had heating pads. These were microwavable little pockets of joy, and my wonderful roommates were great sharers. Whenever I had a time-of-the-month problem or a sore knee or a killer headache, I had full access to heating pad happiness. But after several months of shamelessly hoarding my roommates' heating pads, I decided it was time for me to get my own. After all, having a heating pad is completely essential to womanhood. It's like a warm hug for your uterus.

This was my senior year of college, and I was in full-on denial about the state of my relationship with James. I thought I would ask him to get me a heating pad for my birthday. Normally I'd beat around the bush for a while, pretend that I didn't need anything to be happy. But not this time. Like with the love questionnaire, I really needed that heating pad for this relationship to survive. It was better than asking for a ring, which was beginning to feel less and less like a possibility.

We were in Los Angeles for an improv competition on my birthday weekend, and he'd flown us there free on his flight benefits. I rolled over in our hotel room bed on the morning of my birthday, kissed him, and anticipated my gift.

"What'd ya get me?" I said coyly.

"What do you mean?" He frowned. "I got you here to LA. That's your gift."

"Oh, of course. Right." I turned over. "Thanks, baby."

My birthday passed. No heating pad, not even a card from James. I appreciated being able to use his flight benefits, but at the time I felt cheated. My naive brain had invented the expectation, reasoning that after nearly five years together, he'd have no problem getting a birthday present for his wannabe future wife. Plus, I really needed that fucking heating pad.

I couldn't let it go. When we got back from LA, I suggested we go shopping together to find a heating pad for my birthday. I offered to pay for it too. He was extremely put out by the suggestion.

"Fine, whatever," he said, and pushed past me to the car.

"I'm not trying to be materialistic," I said. "I just thought it would be nice. It can be your gift to me for next Christmas, maybe."

We drove around to a shopping mall and stopped in two stores. He was cold toward me, peeved about the task at hand.

"Look, forget it," I said, choking back tears in an aisle full of pots and pans. "I'm sorry I even asked. Let's just go home."

We drove back to his mom's house in silence. Later I bawled my eyes out over the bathroom sink. It wasn't about the heating pad. I wasn't crying because I didn't get what I wanted, even though the heating pad would have felt great on my heart right about then. I was crying because I felt like I was trapping him; loving me was a chore, something he had to deal with, not enjoy. I never asked for anything again until we exchanged our belongings for the last time only a few months later.

When my brain began to fall apart in August, I received gifts from family members and friends. People didn't know what to make of the fact that my head was leaking, so they'd call up and ask which Disney movies I didn't already own and what my favorite candy was. One day my aunt Diane rang my mother. Mom played it cool as we sat on the couch watching *Just Friends* for the millionth time.

"She's doing all right," she told Aunt Diane. "We're not sure if she'll need surgery or not yet, so we're just waiting."

I crammed a handful of Goldfish into my mouth.

"Sweetheart, do you want to talk to Auntie Di?" she asked. She handed me the receiver as I swallowed crackers that the left side of my tongue couldn't taste.

"Do you need anything, sweetheart?" Aunt Diane asked.

"No, I'm fine, really," I said. "I'm just happy I'm not lesson planning right now."

About a week after that phone call, I received a package from Aunt Diane. It was a heating pad—a *homemade* heating pad. She didn't have a sewing machine, so she'd sewn it up by hand. The material was dark purple with little white flowers dancing around the fabric; it was the most beautiful thing I'd ever seen. It was literally a bag of rice sewn together, but it brought me to tears. Auntie Di had known it would bring me comfort in my pain. She'd done this without being asked. If that's not real love, folks, then I don't know what is.

I sleep with my heating pad every night now. It became routine after rehab to send Brian down to the microwave to heat it as I slowly made my way up to bed. By the time I'd washed my face with one hand while holding on to the sink with the other for dear life, my heating pad was warmed up and ready. Brian would bring it to me as I crawled into bed and swallowed my concoction of steroids and constipation pills.

Mom and Dad would pop their heads into my bedroom. "Do you need any more ice baggies? Hot towel? Yogurt?"

But the answer was always no. I had my heating pad and my handrails. All was right with the world.

### The Great Pumpkin Brain

I've always used current events as costumes. Well, I shouldn't say always. I wasn't exactly dressing up as Monica Lou-in-Skis in 1998. Because I was six years old. But that would have been awesome, even if I was more concerned with how to get the most candy from my kindergarten classmates than I was with the whole scandal.

One Halloween I was Mitt Romney's "binders full of women." Once I was the government shutdown of 2013. If you're wondering how I pulled these costumes off, I offer the photographic proof.

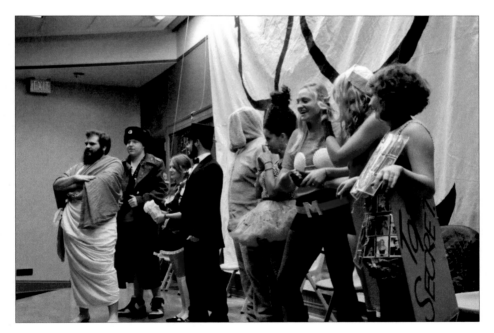

*This is me on the far right as Mitt Romney's "binders full of women," next to Mermaid Man and Barnacle Boy. I won an improv T-shirt for this beauty. Those other chumps didn't stand a chance.*

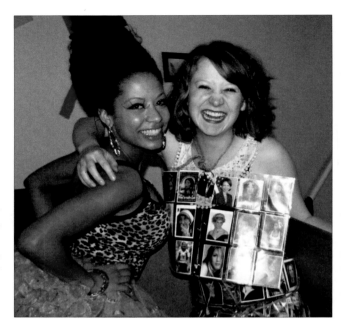

*I would like to point out that this binder full of women includes Princess Diana, Mother Teresa, Condi Rice, and Sacagawea. Because I'm a feminist champion.*

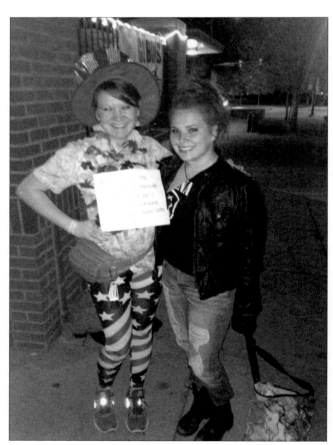

*Me and Scurrboo as the government shutdown of 2013 and some famous rocker chick.*

After a while I began a pattern of political costumes, which is odd, considering how uninvolved I am in politics. It was fun being viewed as witty and well-informed. I felt respected. Well, more respected than, say, a slutty librarian. Or a slutty Supreme Court justice. Slutty anything. Everyone does slutty on Halloween, let's be honest.

People who don't dress up for Halloween are party poopers. Why wouldn't you take advantage of the one holiday where you get to dress like a sexy lampshade and consume bags upon bags of Almond Joys with no shame? Okay…a little bit of shame. But in all fairness, that toilet was just asking to be thrown up in. Listen, I'm not proud of Halloween 2011. Or my birthday 2011. Let's get real, *all* of 2011. But I am quite proud of Halloween 2014.

That year's costume shall live on in notoriety forever, thanks to my architect father and crafty mother. I proposed the idea of the Great Pumpkin Brain at the onset of my illness.

"Just you wait 'til Halloween," I told the nursing staff at my first hospital visit. "My costume's gonna kill it." Well, kill it, it most certainly did.

My dad is a master architect and design genius. My mom has a sewing machine, and I grew up wearing adorable matching mother and daughter outfits. Putting the two of them in a room together with a sick child and a quirky costume concept was like watching an episode of *Project Runway* while you're high.

My mother's plan involved pool noodles. Yes, I did say pool noodles. She wanted to mimic the noodly nature of brain matter and thought that pool floaties were the obvious answer. "Let's get a bunch of gray ones and weave them together like spaghetti!" she said excitedly as my dad hunted online for a deal.

"You guys, I don't need anything fancy. Maybe just a silly T-shirt or something—"

"A T-shirt! We can hold up the pool noodles by sewing them onto a T-shirt!" My mother had those terrifying stars in her eyes that only someone who crafts in the summertime would understand.

It wasn't working. I was only exciting them more. Before I knew it, my dad had hit the Purchase button on an industrial-sized box of jumbo pool noodles, and my mother was unearthing her 1965 Singer from the basement and hauling it into her bedroom.

"You guys, really," I said. "Don't you think this is a *little* excessive?"

My brother snickered. "Go big or go back to rehab, sis."

While Mom awaited the arrival of the precious pool noodles, my dad began a model of his own. Unbeknownst to my mother, he had been quietly drafting a design for days. I heard them arguing about the whole thing late one night.

"No, no, the T-shirt will never hold that weight—"

"But we'll *sew* her into it!"

"But with my foam design, she can slide in and out. We don't need to sew her into anything, dear!"

This conversation lasted for days. It would have lasted longer, had Halloween not been less than a week away. Then the pool noodles came. My mother attempted to take her XXL T-shirt and sew it together with the bazookas. Right as she thought she'd created a masterpiece and won the whole argument, the pool noodle ripped right in half. To make matters more hilarious, she stuffed her head into the ripped pool noodle and paraded around my bedroom like the most spectacular human I'd ever seen. Dad's foam design would win this fight. But at least Mom wasn't a sore loser.

Dad and Brian went to the hardware store to find the "brain foam." When they plopped it down in the living room that evening, I inspected the rectangular brick uneasily. It looked like that heavy-duty insulation you find in old attics. And in padded hospital rooms.

"Is this…my costume?" I said.

"It will be!" Dad flashed his big up-to-no-good grin.

For the next twelve hours I heard him banging about in the garage as he glued the gigantic pieces together and sliced and diced them with the turkey carver, which I thought was pretty on brand for the whole thing. My parents were putting so much time into the damn costume, I was starting to feel like the crazy one. How had they taken me seriously in the first place? Wasn't everything that came out of my mouth ridiculous sarcasm?

After an hour or so Dad wheeled in his brain-shaped pièce de résistance.

Now, before I show you the pictures, know that this thing was massive. It was ridiculously detailed. And it actually resembled a brain. Like spot-on, *holy shit, Dad, who knew you could make a hunk of foam look like that with the turkey carver?* There were grooves in it that made it look like actual brain matter. *Jesus, Dad. Take it down a notch. Or twelve.*

"Where do I fit?" I eyed the apparatus with doubt.

He flipped it upward to reveal a human-shaped hole in the center for me to squeeze into. His grin was so huge, it almost bounced off his jolly face.

I put my arms up as he tried to squish the brainy foam onto my body. No luck. Damn you, normal-sized boobs.

"A little bigger, Dad."

He ran off to the garage with the electric turkey carver to make the hole bigger. He didn't want it too big; it was built to sit on my huge hips. No sewing or straps needed.

After several small adjustments, we squished the thing comfortably onto my body, and I took it for a spin around the kitchen. It was wobbly and fabulous. Walking in it was a physical therapy exercise in itself. All that was needed now was the paint job, and two cans of dark gray spray paint later, the garage was left smelling of the best costume of all time. Dad took bits of red paint and splattered them around to show the blood vessels.

But it wasn't finished yet. Mom accepted defeat now that the foam design had won, but she sewed up a large Band-Aid with the word "Ouch!" to be placed directly at my injury site, or on my costume, my ass. It was glorious. My parents had successfully made me into a real-life brain, ready to wreak havoc anywhere I went.

My destination of choice? Pearl Street in Boulder, the biggest pub crawl in Colorado during the witching hour. Never mind that I wasn't allowed to drink alcohol yet. It didn't matter. I was going to have the best costume in the whole city.

But before I took the Great Pumpkin Brain down Pearl, I brought it to therapy. The therapists were sure to get a fucking kick out of this one.

I sauntered into the main office. "Hello, I believe I'm scheduled for some jump-rope activities this morning…"

"You have got to be kidding me…Jen, Vicki, everyone, get over here!" the nurse at the station yelled down the hall.

It didn't take long for the Great Pumpkin Brain to go viral at Spalding. I puttered around the hospital in between my workouts, slipping the brain on and off my hips to check in on various patients or to hand out Halloween stickers. Just your usual brain stuff.

By the time my therapy session was up, I was snapping pictures with every employee in the place and feeling like Justin Bieber on a Canadian tour.

"Mimi, where are you going with that thing tonight? To the bars? You know the doc says you can't drink yet…"

"Yeah, I know. Who cares? Do you know how many dudes I'm going to pick up tonight with this big…cerebellum?!"

Approximately five. That's how many. And at least thirty compliments on my Band-Aid.

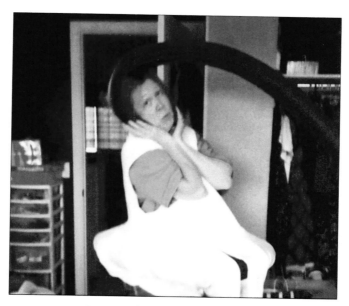

*Mom modeling the first prototype.*

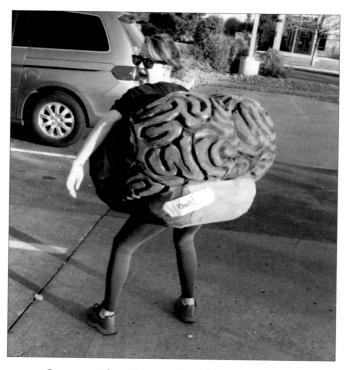

*Stranger at bar: Dang, girl, yo' brain is hugeeeee.*
*Me: *twerks* My safe word is cerebral cortex.*

### License to *Tokyo Drift*

Everybody says old people shouldn't drive. And an old lady did nearly send me sailing off a cliff the other day. But nobody understands why they get so grumpy when we take away their keys.

"Don't be ridiculous, Grandma! Why are you getting upset? Do you want to cause a five-car pileup?"

We call our decision to shred their licenses and hide their keys a public service and move along down the freeway. But did we ever stop to think that when we do that, we are taking away their independence too?

I realized this after being told I couldn't drive due to my double vision. Well, duh. I was obviously too sick to go to the Saturday night raves with my college buds, but part of me still thought that I could. During the six weeks of bedrest and uncertainty before my surgery, I had full intentions of running a half marathon, learning how to cook, and vacationing in the south of France. I never considered that I couldn't do these things until I was specifically told that I couldn't. Until I was told no to the things I'd been doing for years. I felt like I was going backward instead of forward in my life. I had a college degree but nowhere to take it.

Fortunately for me, I can still do all these things. Even if the vacationing in southern France does seem a bit out of my price range at the moment. I am young and resilient, and my fast-paced recovery from brain trauma reflects that. But to an elderly person, being told you can't do something can be like a death sentence. If a young person gets in a car accident and can't go fishing for a while, no big deal. They'll be back at it in no time. But when Grandpa has a stroke and is told he'll never fish again, you feel his pain. You feel it in his eyes and in his soul.

I met some truly beautiful people during my rehabilitation, many of whom were fifty to sixty years older than I was. They had lived unbelievable lives, and they shared their experiences with me so openly and honestly that it makes me cry even now. Here I was, some silly twenty-two-year-old complaining about heartbreak, when they had seen wars, built families and lost them, and worked incredibly hard to survive. I was such a life rookie. I hadn't done anything to survive; I hadn't worked up a sweat to make a living or support a loved one. But they had, and they taught me lessons about the world that I had never learned in school or read in a book. Really, the only way to know how to live is to talk to someone who has. These people had *lived* things, *seen* things, and I was honored to know them, even for a short while. Hearing about their struggles to get back to their old lives before injury humbled me. I was one of the lucky ones; I was quickly getting back to the old me and all the little pieces of independence that came with it.

The day I got my license back was a special day. I mean, they hadn't exactly taken it away. They'd just highly advised me not to take the family car out on a joyride to Dairy Queen. I was fine with this, considering I could always play the brain card and make one of my friends go and get me the Dairy Queen anyway.

Since leaving Spalding inpatient therapy, I'd been going back three days a week for a few hours of PT and OT on the outpatient floor. I'd upgraded from wheelchair to hot wheels in a few short months. Now I reflected back on the days when people didn't trust me to go to the bathroom on my own, much less take the good ol' Cruiser out for an excursion.

But I was still nervous. The tape on my glasses had gotten smaller and smaller, until we'd finally taken it off when I could see singular again. I didn't know, though, if my vision was good enough to distinguish all the signs on the road. And what if I jerked my head around and got dizzy? What if the red lights looked like green lights? Whose nice Mercedes would I pile into then?

My new occupational therapist, Jen, outlined the precautions for brain-injured motorists. "You need to check those mirrors," she said. "And try not to turn your head too fast when you look at those blind spots."

My neck mobility had improved greatly, but I still experienced dizziness if I turned my head too quickly. The lingering issue was the vision—which was kind of necessary for driving. Jen and I had been doing light sensor tests all week to prepare me for a checkup with my ophthalmologist, an eye doctor who specializes in the brain's connection with the eye. Also a word I'm sure I'll never be able to pronounce.

A large black lightboard, five feet by five feet and covered in tiny holes, stretched across a wall in the exercise gym. Jen would pick a speed, and one by one the lights would flicker on in various holes around the board. My task was to stand in front and touch the lights as fast as I could. From this test, they'd be able to tell which fields of vision were my weakest and whether I'd be ready to drive again soon.

My fancy eye doctor came in later that day for more tests, flashing weird lights in my eyes and asking me to read letters off a chart as he moved it swiftly up and down. The most impressive test was a laser beam that he shot directly into my eyeball, making lines of light appear across my peripheral vision.

"Can I keep one of these?" I said, motioning to an eye patch in his kit as he shot another laser beam at my retina.

"Of course!" he said. "But I doubt you'll need one with these eyes! They're looking great. Jen, she's good to drive anytime she wants."

I did a happy dance in my chair, excited to drive myself places like a real grown-up. Maybe I'd go get ice cream. Or to the store to buy a nice pair of dancing shoes. Or both! The possibilities were endless.

When I got home from therapy, I made sure to text all my friends in Boulder, alerting them that I was ready to party. I asked Mom if I could drive us to our pottery class. To keep me from becoming bored out of my mind, she had enrolled us in a group class, and I knew she was excited to see me being creative again. Or maybe she hoped that taking my frustration out on lumps of clay would be more productive than other activities, like crying in my bedroom or watching more Bruce Willis flicks.

"Easy getting out of the garage!" she cautioned me now as I rolled her Tahoe gently down the driveway.

"Mom, I got this," I said. "I've driven a car before."

"Check your mirrors!" she screamed. "Do you need help parking?"

It was like I was sixteen all over again. Mom with her "oh *shit*" handle and phantom brake pedal that she'd occasionally step on as I neared a stoplight. Her nerves oozed over from the passenger side.

As we drove down the street, I glanced at the moving autumn leaves. I tried not to watch them too much; their motion made me dizzy. My latest physical therapy exercise with my new therapist, Sylvia, was walking on a treadmill and looking in different directions. It had seemed trivial at the time, but now I saw how it had been preparing me for this moment in the car.

"Careful!" Mom shouted. "Corner!"

"They have corners on this street now?" I laughed. "I had no idea. I must have been gone a long time."

Mom did not indulge my tomfoolery.

I chuckled to Dad when we got home that we'd barely made it alive down the two blocks to the pottery studio. My mother collapsed on the couch in exhaustion. I was tired too, from being so upright and alert. But it was good to take baby steps again.

Of course, I wanted to wrap a scarf around my head and let it blow in the wind down the highway. But I needed to get to know the driveway first.

I was lucky to have my independence back, unlike others in my situation. Even if I was upset that I didn't qualify for a handicapped parking sticker. That was the biggest tragedy of all. I had my license and my freedom back, and I was ready to *Tokyo Drift*. I could resume the activities I'd done before my ailment, with only minor precautions now. I could drive myself to therapy and stop for a cheeseburger on the way home and actually taste it. I could carry lightweight boxes around the house without fear of tumbling down the stairs and breaking my face and head open again.

I could even plan a lesson for my return to teaching in January, if I wanted to. Which I really didn't.

# Napkin Notes

"Good morning, baby! Have a wonderful day! I LOVE YOU."

I scribbled the words and a giant smiley face with curly hair onto the back of a Chipotle receipt and slid it mischievously into James's wallet.

This was roughly a year before I'd come to terms with the fact that I never wanted James to have a wonderful day again. But at the time, I was content scribbling love notes on every surface of his mother's apartment until he said something about it. He never did. Love notes just "weren't his thing anymore."

They were mine. I love leaving notes for people. It's my ultimate favorite. I enjoy smothering loved ones with doodles, adorable to-do lists, and the occasional haiku. And who doesn't like finding a sticky note on their car that they instantly mistake for a parking ticket?

Sometimes people acknowledge my notes. Sometimes they think they're a little weird and random. Sometimes they're right about that, but we'll get to that part in a bit.

I was two months into my post-rehab recovery now, and I could only leave so many love notes for my mother before she grew concerned for my well-being. To keep me from crafting tiny Christmas angels made of garden pots for the fifth day in a row, she suggested I go up to Boulder to see my college buddies. Lexi and her boyfriend, Peter, were putting on a comedy show that weekend.

Naturally I wrote Lexi a "break a leg" letter on a napkin and tucked it in my pocket for later. "Hey, y'all," I said, sneaking backstage during their rehearsal. "Snacks are here!"

"Scurrrrrrr…" Lexi squealed from the corner of the room.

"BOO!" Don't ask me what this means. I have no idea. It's just what we've called each other since college.

"Got you something." I unearthed the dirty napkin from my pocket, and she set down her stage makeup.

"A napkin note? Nope, not reading it 'til after the show. I don't need to be crying in this beard right now."

I hugged her tightly and allowed her and the crew to finish rehearsal.

The show was amazing, satirical sketches interwoven with the theme of YouTube

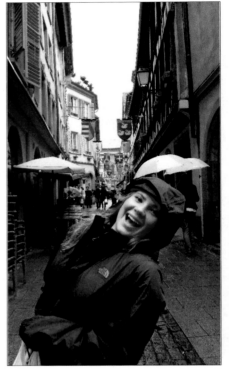

*My personal favorite picture of my Scurrboo from that time we ran around three countries in two days.*

and social media. Lexi played a bearded pope, and our friend Wade cross-dressed as a jealous girlfriend. I loved every minute of it. Lexi had earned her napkin note.

Later that night, I wrote a second napkin note. This note was received by a bearded god. The beard was real. And the man attached to it was surely made by heaven.

After the show, Lexi and I walked to our favorite sandwich bar; it was our tradition after shows to grab a pint and split a footlong. She spotted a friend at a table in the back. "Hey, Chris!"

I was not interested in Chris. Sitting at this friend's table was the most beautiful man I had ever laid my now-functioning eyeballs on.

I made eye contact, shook his gorgeous hand, and mumbled something about improv. He seemed like he was listening, which was a good start. It was last call, though, so we had to hurry to order our sandwiches and beer. Lexi and I ended up at a table an unfortunately good distance from the stunning man. I awkwardly stared at him from across the bar.

"Why is your face doing that?" Lexi said.

"Doing what?" I said as I ogled him more.

"Your *face*," she whispered. "*Stop that.*" Apparently I was making an undoubtedly ugly face while staring at his beautiful one. I suppose I was astonished that someone this good-looking could live in the same universe. *That guy is way out of my league,* I thought. *What would he want with some bumbling, brain-damaged chick?* Lexi read my mind like an open issue of *Cosmo* and ripped off a piece of napkin.

"What am I supposed to do with this?" I asked. I'd already written her a napkin note before the show.

"Put your number on it, you dummy," Lexi said through bites of eggplant.

Out of the corner of my eye, I saw Sir Naughty Lips get up with his friends to leave. So I panicked. Lexi gave me the "it's go time, girl" face and whipped out a pen—presumably from her ass—and I scrambled to write down my number just as he exited the bar. I made a mad dash toward him and slipped on a puddle. He was already outside with his friends when I reached him, holding out the note.

"You dropped this!" I said, uncomfortably loud.

I threw the napkin at his face before he could make eye contact with my crazy pupils. Then I sprinted back into the bar like a goddamn champion.

I was totally off my game. That is, if I'd ever had game in the first place. How could I be so completely un-smooth? If that handsome guy was James Bond, then I was Pee Wee Herman. A Bond girl would have known better. A Bond girl wouldn't have had to say anything. She would have given him the sexy eyes from a mile away, and Bond would have come running. My sexy eyes consisted of a lot of blinking, a contact falling out of my eyeball, and me scrambling on the floor to look for it.

Lexi called me a brave, ballsy soul, and we finished our sandwiches and chugged our beer before they kicked us out to shut down the bar. We decided to keep barhopping in hopes that I'd find another gorgeous gentleman to humiliate myself in front of.

By then most of the other bars were closing too. We'd just barely made it to the Downer when they announced last call. *Perfect timing*, I thought. Then I saw Handsome McGee.

"Shitshitshitshitshit!" I said out loud. Lexi traced my line of sight, and her face lit up like the sun on steroids. She dragged me down to the bar.

"No, please," I begged. "It's Napkin Man."

She walked right up to him and thrust the two of us together. My face went head-on into his chest plate like a torpedo.

"Hi, sorry," I said, recovering from what seemed like another traumatic head injury. "I don't know her." I shot Lexi death daggers through my eye sockets.

"You're Mimi, right?" he asked.

"Yeah," I said. "Listen, I'm sorry about the whole––"

"No problem," he said. "Come sit with us." He ushered me over to a table with the rest of his friends. Lexi gave me a thumbs-up. I felt like I'd entered the twilight zone.

Napkin Man and I sat and talked for the remaining time the bar was open, which sadly was only about fifteen minutes. He told me he was a mathematics student going for his master's degree. I swooned. He told me he was thinking about being a high school teacher. I drooled. Then he said he liked improv. I just about had a fucking heart attack. He didn't even seem terribly creeped out by my napkin-throwing ways, or at least he didn't show it. I thought he was too good to be true.

In my mind I thanked him for talking to me, because I was just a lowly peasant and he was a powerful and beautifully bearded god from above who had obviously stooped to converse with me. We stepped out of the bar, and I reunited with my friends and he with his.

"See?" Lexi slurred. "Aren't I such a gooD wink WOman?"

"You're drunk," I said. "Let's go home, *wink woman*."

I relayed my conversation with the supermodel/god to her as we stopped for a grilled cheese at a nearby food cart. I had a feeling my scents of Crazy and Desperate had surely made a stink of the place, scaring him away from me forever. These were no Calvin Klein's Unforgettably Sexy, but they were all I had at the moment, okay?

When we got into our Uber, I made matters even more awkward, as if that was possible. I Facebook-stalked him. I did this because in addition to being insane, I am wise enough to realize that technology is a Christmas miracle that saves lives and ruins future relationships. I also thought it was the end of the world and that I would never see him again because he was going on the *Apollo 14* mission to destroy an asteroid. Yes, even after having my brain operated on, I managed to have an overactive imagination gland.

Unfortunately I found him on Facebook.

I knew friending him would be a death sentence. So instead I went for a double death sentence. Or, to put it visually, I hurled my body off the Empire State Building and then power-washed my remaining body parts into the gutter. This is the message I sent to the beautiful Napkin Man:

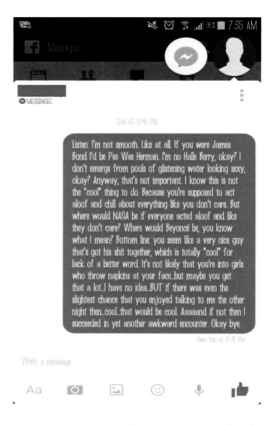

Listen: I'm not smooth. Like at all. If you were James Bond I'd be Pee Wee Herman. I'm no Halle Berry, okay? I don't emerge from pools of glistening water looking sexy, okay? Anyway, that's not important. I know this is not the "cool" thing to do. Because you're supposed to act aloof and chill about everything like you don't care. But where would NASA be if everyone acted aloof and like they don't care? Where would Beyoncé be, you know what I mean? Bottom line: you seem like a very nice guy that's got his shit together, which is totally "cool" for lack of a better word. It's not likely that you're into girls who throw napkins at your face...but maybe you get that a lot. I have no idea...BUT if there was even the slightest chance that you enjoyed talking to me the other night then...cool...that would be cool. Aaaaand if not then I succeeded in yet another awkward encounter. Okay bye.

As you can see, the message was seen about sixty seconds after I sent it. Being an undoubtedly sane person, he did not respond. Was I surprised? Of course not. I will admit that I come off strong. But so does scotch, and plenty of rich people drink that.

"Did you really just send that?" Lexi asked, eyeing my phone.

"I mean, it's not the best life policy," I said. "But if my future self doesn't bust down the door and prevent me from doing it, then how bad can it be, really?"

I wanted to know what it was like to take a risk again. I wanted to throw myself helplessly into a nonexistent love affair. Instead I was falling back into the same brain waves as before. To me, I was being brave and ambitious. I thought I was getting back in the saddle. But this time I wasn't riding the slow-motion bull that Vicki and I had practiced with in rehab. It was a full-blown, super-speed, bucking longhorn. And I was careening to the pavement without a helmet strapped to my heart.

# How to Be Rejected by a Canadian

There is a stereotype for everyone. There is a stereotype for mail carriers, golf ball collectors, and people who "don't like chocolate." Also for the mother of the bride and cat people. Stereotypes are a way for our brains to bring order to an order-less world or even protect us. Because I was nearly run off the road today by a Prius and a middle finger, my brain might tell me that all Prius owners are reckless and out to kill me. And maybe they are.

As someone with French Canadian origins, I am aware of the stereotypes for Canadians, eh? Hockey-playing, snow-shoveling, and so nice that people want to punch them in the face; these are just a few we all know and love.

When I revisited online dating after recovery, I found a Canadian. To be clear, he was living in Denver at the time. This wasn't some sketchy "oh, we're getting married in June, but I've never actually met the guy" kind of love. To be even clearer, it wasn't love at all. It was just a date. A first date with dim lighting and a bowl of guacamole made right in front of our eyes by Quinn, my personal guacamole maker.

I used to like first dates. Aside from having my face held by a future serial killer, I quite enjoyed being courted by men. Now I equate first dates to agonizing, alcohol-induced interviews. And not the interview for being the first human on Mars, which is the job you *really* want. No. It's an interview for Papa John's. And while I do enjoy pizza, I do not enjoy wearing off-yellow uniforms and standing behind sneeze guards.

The date starts out with an attempt to find the most appropriate and non-awkward way to greet each other. This is usually a handshake that shrivels into a passive-aggressive hug, but if you're a serial killer, you can also hold your date's face and stare into their eyeballs. Then you spend the next three hours talking about boring subjects while simultaneously trying to stuff your face without looking like a wildebeest. Who in the hell cares about my glory days in high school sports? Who in the hell cares about which brand of cereal I prefer? I mean, I do. But even then, I don't really. Just hearing myself talk about me feels so alien and wrong. And that is why alcohol exists.

The worst part about a first date is when you realize after the first thirty seconds of meeting them that you made a horrible mistake. Then you must endure the interview process at least until your guac arrives, and that could be an entire half hour from now, depending on how quickly you get Quinn's attention.

Canada, the person I went on the date with, not the country, was not the Papa John's interview. I thought he was NASA. He was cute and charming and a petroleum engineer. I blabbered on and on about my silly brain and downed two margaritas before I even discussed my stint in rehab. This was my first date since my brain injury, and I was excited to make use of my safe word. But I didn't want to hide who I really was.

"Would you like some more chips for your guacamole?" Quinn asked.

"Why, yes, Quinn, we would like that very much," I said. Canada was impressed that Quinn and I were on a first-name basis. Little did he know that I'd gotten to the date twenty minutes early, taken a nervous pre-date poop, and then made friends with the guacamole guy.

Canada and I sat with our guacamole for a few hours, talking and laughing. He was handsome and charismatic. But I can honestly say I didn't learn much about him that night. I was so focused on landing the interview to go to Mars that I missed out on the opportunity to ask NASA some questions. What's space food really like? What if I don't like my astronaut colleagues? *Where does the poop go?*

He walked me out of the restaurant, and we parted ways with a metaphorical *poof.* He was only in town for a few more days, so for the next two months we talked vaguely and sporadically via text—me in Colorado, him in Canada. A natural love story.

You know how some people wear their heart on their sleeve? I wear my heart on my face. Right on my goddamn forehead. I quickly invented ways for me and my Canadian pal to date long distance. I even wrote the guy a fucking letter. On a piece of paper. And I put it in the mailbox *with a Canadian postage stamp.* He got it three weeks later and said he liked it. I also sent him clips of me playing songs on the guitar, and I don't even play guitar. That's how much of a crazy lunatic I am. *Wanna go on a first date?*

After months of awkwardly exchanging vague (or not so vague on my end) "I like you" texts, I was finally visited by the Angel of Budding Future Relationships. In five days we'd both be at the Los Angeles airport at the same time, me for an improv festival at the University of Southern California and him for a layover on his way to San Diego for a family trip. What an opportunity! What a great way to meet up with my nonexistent love interest! That is, until he updated his Facebook page that he was in a relationship. And not with me. Well, shit.

I'd played this all up in my stupid, gooey brain again. For two months I'd wholeheartedly convinced myself that what the Canadian and I had was real. I'd gone on one date with the guy. He lived in another country. Had my brain surgery done anything at all to fix my screwed-up delusions?

They'd gone in to fix what was wrong with me. But I already knew—*I* was wrong with me. I'd spent the last five years of my life dragging myself down. I'd wired my brain around James, who was surely gone now after my subtle text reply back at Spalding, and my brain was already hard at work rewiring the system. Of course, I'd gone about it in all the wrong ways. I'd thrown myself back into dating so that I wouldn't have to face myself—so that I wouldn't have to look at my reflection in the mirror and realize that I was messed up.

While I would have appreciated a "hey, I'm not interested, found somebody else" text from the Canadian, I acknowledge that there's not always time for that. We move through life at such a fast pace that we sometimes cut people off on the freeway by accident. And sometimes genuine romantic feelings are easily confused with, well, being Canadian, if you buy into the stereotype. He made an apology after I went full-out Taylor Swift on him and threatened to write him into my book as another degenerate. I threw my hands up in quasi-forgiveness.

*You know you could have told me, right, bro?* But how could I expect anyone to tell me the truth if I was unwilling to hear it from myself?

# I'm Peeing as We Sleep

You may recall a previous chapter entitled "I'm Peeing as We Speak." Fear not, good friends. This is neither a duplicate chapter nor a mistake in the editing room. And like much of this book, this chapter is not advised for the weak of heart or stomach. Or my mother. Or my future boyfriend. I'd rather the two of you just skipped this chapter, actually.

I currently hold the record for the worst 2014 ever. At least of all the people I've interviewed. I had my heart massacred and I survived massive brain trauma in the span of several months. My friends landed adult jobs and got married while I gazed out the window of a hospital, watching the fall leaves drop. I felt alone, misunderstood, and weak for much of that year. So I did what many people do on New Year's Eve: I decided to get stupid drunk and leave 2014 in the dust, never to be seen or heard from again.

My best friend, Riley, was game to make my New Year's Eve dreams come true. We started our evening at my favorite downtown hipster spot, where I ordered a fancy crab hors d'oeuvre and Riley picked an apple pie dessert.

"You're not allergic to crab, are you?" I asked as a plate of whole crab claws arrived. We'd scoped out the open seating on the roof and somehow managed to land ourselves a nice booth.

"I am," she said. "And you ask me that at least once a month."

"I know." I pointed to my head. "Brain damage. But at least I wore sensible shoes."

"You'd be dead in two minutes on that ice in heels, Miss Brain Damage."

I tucked the crab claws into my sleeves. "Do you notice anything weird about my hands?" I asked. "I don't know, there's just something different about them today." Riley and I snorted. 2015 was off to a great start.

Once we finished the crab claws and pie crusts, we headed down to a place called Beauty Bar to meet up with some of Riley's work friends. Riley drove my car so that she could get used to driving it on ice. Also because I planned on getting white girl wasted later in the evening. My hot doctor had cleared me to drink alcohol, and now I was cashing in and ready to make huge mistakes.

It took us a while to find a parking spot in the area. We had to walk several blocks in subzero temperatures to the bar, then stood in line for half an hour to pay the cover. By the time we got inside, my nose was dripping, and the snot was almost frozen. But when we discovered the open bar, it took me all of five seconds to discard my coat and squeeze myself to the front. There Riley introduced me to her work friend, Carly.

We hustled our rum and Cokes to the corner of the dance floor and began dancing our faces off. The disco ball made us look fabulous, I thought. I got down with my bad self. I even started freestyle rapping. I was drunk enough to make people believe I knew how to twerk but not enough to ignore the fact that my sequined dress was scratching the inside of my arms like a pissed-off kitten.

Just as I considered asking the bartender for some Band-Aids for my bleeding arms, the moment came that we had all been waiting for: the countdown to the new year. A projector displayed a colorful countdown from ten, and I shouted along at the top of my lungs. It was time. Time for me to leave a miserable year behind and start anew.

On New Year's Eve everyone thinks time works in mystical ways. It's as if we believe that on December 31, history will suddenly erase itself and we can write a new story. Pay no mind to that raging hangover, the stranger in the bathtub, or the personal belongings scattered across the Denver metro area. On January 1, we imagine ourselves as completely different people: clean, thin, and happy. We go to the gym for the first time in 365 days and temporarily forget our foibles, lack of income, and inability to run anything under a thirteen-minute mile. We think we are different people, so we set high and unobtainable goals.

Don't get me wrong—I love making goals. And writing lists of goals that have lists underneath them, outlining which steps to take to achieve them. But I'm just telling it like it is: New Year's resolutions don't change us, we change us. We can't erase our past, and we can't undo our mistakes. Our baggage isn't going anywhere, folks. If anything, it's been permanently chained to our cute little ankles. And that's true no matter what day of the year it is.

On December 31, 2014, I thought I could forget my past. I wanted to be a different person, someone who hadn't lost her first love, who didn't have a scar on the back of her head with funky hairs growing around it. Maybe someone who was a few inches taller would be nice too; someone with less frizzy hair. But just as I had decided to be someone else for real, 2015 brought me down a peg.

The jolly-romping in the bar tapered down, and our group of friends headed to Carly's house nearby. Riley and I were too drunk and tired to drive home, so Carly offered to let us stay the night. She was a delightful host, despite our ridiculous behavior, and cooked us munchies and gave us clothes to sleep in. We passed out immediately in her bed, and she took the couch. I slept like a champion. That is, until the *incident*.

Let me preface this part: this is not the me I have ever been nor ever intended to be. As a child, I envisioned myself a graceful adult who could conquer any obstacle and who didn't have adult acne. I'm really embarrassed that we're even talking about this. But since I have been nothing but straightforward, honest, and offensive for the entirety of this book, why turn back now? #YOLO, am I right?

*Gulp.* Sorry, Mom.

I woke up about five in the morning in Carly's bed on January 1, 2015. It was dark and cold, and I couldn't understand why. I mean, I knew how I'd gotten there, but I didn't know why I was so cold. I felt around the bed and gasped out loud. I was soaking wet—and so was the bed. At first I prayed that I had somehow impaled myself on a bedpost and was slowly bleeding all over the place. Maybe another nurse had dumped an IV bag in my lap again. I prayed for this because it would have been much less embarrassing than the truth.

Which was that I had pissed in the bed. In my drunken sleep. I'd awoken in the new year of 2015, a year that was supposed to be filled with promise, covered in my own piss in a stranger's bed. *What the actual fuck.*

In the seconds following my arrival at this truth, I convinced myself that nobody would notice. Maybe by the time everyone woke up, it would have dried, and I could pretend this had never happened. After all, where had all this urine come from? I'd stopped drinking hours ago. I'd gone to the bathroom immediately before bed.

I tried to inch myself away from my shame and fall asleep.

That's when Riley stirred next to me. She sat up in bed and started feeling around, as I had. I could see her eyes piercing the darkness of the room.

"Dude, are you okay?" Riley whispered.

"Dude, no," I said. "I think I just pissed in her bed." To this day I don't know how I said it with a straight face. "What do I do?"

"We need to wake Carly up," she said. The words were a death sentence. Never in my life had I thought I'd find myself here—shaking a stranger awake and explaining to them that I'd peed in their bed. I stumbled over to the couch and did it anyway.

"Okay," she mumbled. "That's fine."

"I'm really sorry."

Riley helped me grab the sheets and blankets and clothes. "We'll be back later," she told Carly.

Then came the most shameful walk of shame ever to shame the shameful walls of the Wall of Shame. *Shameshameshame.*

We left Carly's apartment with the bundle of urine-soaked sheets. It was five thirty and well below freezing. I held the bundle tight to my chest as we walked, trying to ignore the stench and the way my own piss kept me warm from the cold. I wasn't ready to laugh at myself yet. My teeth chattered relentlessly as Riley and I made our way back to the car.

Once we got to Riley's place, she threw the shame into the washing machine and gave me clean clothes to sleep in.

"I promise I won't piss in your bed too," I said as we crawled under the covers.

"I know," Riley said.

We got up a few hours later, and I came to terms with reality. After we switched the sheets from the washer to the dryer, I went to the grocery store to grab some "I'm sorry for pissing in your bed" bagels for Carly. That didn't feel like enough, so I also bought an "I'm sorry for pissing in your bed" potted plant. When we got back to Carly's apartment, I delivered her gifts and cleaned sheets. I tried my best to look her in the eye.

"Seriously," she said, laughing. "It's okay."

"It's really not," I said.

"My ex-husband used to do that all the time." She set her cup of coffee on the counter. "And he wasn't even drunk."

We left Carly's, and I laughed at myself then, and all morning and well into the afternoon. Come to mention it, I'm still laughing. I'm certainly not proud of this moment, and relaying the ridiculous story in hopes that we remain friends and that you continue to read this book is a risk I'm not entirely sure I should take.

But there you have it. I rang in the new year by peeing in a stranger's bed. I tried to forget James and my brain and all the hurt I'd gone through in the past year. I tried to suppress my harrowing experiences on the exercise balls in rehab. I turned my back on myself and was smacked directly in the face by 2015. That has been the definition of my life so far. Just a two-by-four to the forehead.

We can't run from our lives. I know that now. And New Year's can't solve our problems, just like walking around the block can't cure a brain hemorrhage. When we want change, we have to make it for ourselves. We must own our lives and our stories every single day—the good, the bad, and the piss-covered sheets. And first we must confront our truest (and sometimes disgusting) selves, clean those sheets, and move on with our lives the best we can.

Mom, if you're still there, again I am *sorrrryyyyyyyy*.

# My Therapists Probably Think I'm Dead by Now

"We're going to need eighty-five double-sided copies of the Syria maps and then a class set of thirty questions..." Lindsay said as I scribbled the information onto a miniature sticky note. I adjusted the phone and twirled the pen in my hand.

"Got it," I said. "And seating charts, and bulletin boards decorated, and I'll go buy us more coffee." The coffee was the most important thing. I could drink that again without my heart exploding. I'd need as much of it as possible to get through today and the next six months.

Christmas break was over, as was my vacation from real adult responsibility. The past few months had skewed my sense of reality. They'd made me think I could nap whenever I wanted and tune out the loud world with Claude Debussy if I got stressed out. But it was back to business now and a chance for a fresh start. Or another fresh start after my smelly NYE debacle.

As far as I was concerned, my brain injury had never happened. There wouldn't be room for it in the packed high school hallways. It was a thing of yesteryear, an illusion that I told myself was from a past life—a historical event that I could explain to students dispassionately. Even my brain book ventures had gone to hell in a colorful handbasket. As the reality of the upcoming semester crashed in around me like the trash compactor in *Star Wars*, I exchanged my writing for lesson planning in eight-hour increments and spewing the entire contents of my teacher bag across my parents' living room.

I was scared out of my fucking mind.

I hung up the phone with Lindsay and placed the sticky note in my blue leather notebook, the one with "Enjoy Every Moment" on the front cover. I'd bought it back in August for my student teaching semester to remind me to enjoy the challenging parts of teaching too. But so much had happened since I'd purchased that little blue notebook in the bookstore across the street from the high school. I clung to the notebook now and questioned if it could miraculously rescue me from a second brain rupture.

I eyed my to-do list. Why were there so many items? Why couldn't I remember how to do them? What did *SLO* stand for again? The words seemed to ooze over and on top of each other, and I recalled my double vision, when everything spread apart and multiplied. Now things were coming back together, but too fast. My eyes were fine. But my head was not.

During outpatient therapy at Spalding, Jen had tasked me with creating and teaching a lesson I could use once I got back to school. It was mid-November then, and three more teenage boys had joined the hospital gang. I thought they'd make the perfect guinea pigs.

I went home and stared at my blank screen for a few days. With unlimited time to lesson plan, I was supposed to be coming up with Hilary Swank material. I was supposed to be delivering like Robin Williams. Back in college I'd taken a course on the American Pilgrims and their interactions with Native Americans. I looked through my old college books and decided to work one into the lesson for Jen and the brain buds. I called my lesson "The Real Thanksgiving," hoping that giving it a name might mask the fact that I had no idea what I was doing.

The day of the lesson, I set up my PowerPoint in the conference room and made copies of my reading. I carefully connected my computer to the projector and meticulously laid out readings at each seat around the conference table before my students arrived.

"Welcome, everyone!" I smiled brightly as they entered the room. A few of the first-floor therapists who were on break had joined us as well. "Today we're going to learn about the real Thanksgiving," I said. I hit the Next button on my computer like I was the best there ever was. Youngblood flashed an approving thumbs-up as I switched slides.

What I hadn't anticipated was how ill-suited my readings were to my mainly sixteen-year-old audience. The readings came from a college-level novel from a history class. Its language was thick and hard to understand. Even I couldn't comprehend what I was talking about. Let's not even mention the fact that we all had fucking head injuries and could barely read in the first place.

My slides were crowded with too much information. The readings didn't make sense, and no one knew what kind of notes they were supposed to be taking. I was starting to lose my audience, so I paused the slideshow and improvised. I asked Youngblood if he'd learned anything new about Thanksgiving since we'd started our lesson.

"I didn't know about the crazy things people did before," he said. "Now I think it's a lot more complicated than just eating a bunch of turkey and watching football."

My timer sounded, and my fifty-minute lesson was over. I exhaled. Everyone clapped. I gathered my papers and shut down my presentation, feeling silly about playing teacher for an hour. I was so out of practice. But then again, I was never really in practice. My dramatic brain bleed had made damn sure of that.

As I began a mental narrative of the potential failure of my future teaching career, Youngblood shuffled up to me on his crutches. He'd recently upgraded from the wheelchair. "Hey!" he said. "You did a great job. You're going to be an awesome teacher someday." He smiled at me, and my heart warmed up.

I'd known then deep down that he was right. But here I was now, just as nervous as when I'd started that practice lesson. I stood in the kitchen as Mom prodded me for a second attempt at a first day of school picture. Hopefully this time I'd survive past my first week.

"Beautiful!" Mom gushed as we reviewed the selfie. "You look beautiful. You're going to do amazing."

And when I stepped out of my car in the parking lot at East High, I was happy. Happier than I'd been in, shit, probably a year. I looked up at the building just as I had before. Despite my own radical transformation, it remained the same, solid and unchanged. This was a major source of relief. I dusted off my pencil skirt for bagel crumbs and made my way through the gleaming double doors.

When my students arrived for my fourth period class, they applauded me. These were the kids who'd written me get-well cards and asked about my return for the last three months. It was like a scene from a movie. And I was the hero.

"Welcome back, Ms. H!" they shouted. Bruce Willis clapped his approval from my shoulder. *Way to go, kid.*

Save your applause, everyone. No really. Save it. I'm going to bed at five o'clock, so you need to keep it down, because I'm fucking exhausted.

~

Teaching proved harder than ever that spring. It was hard because it was teaching. But it was harder because it was teaching with a brain injury. Sometimes I was confident in my ability to plan and deliver lessons for the kids, but other days left me breathless and panicked.

At school I couldn't control my environment. One day I dressed in too many layers and became overheated during class. I ripped off my layers, only to realize that I still couldn't breathe. Lindsay sent me away to get some air, and I walked into the courtyard to allow the chilly air to hit my lungs. The quiet of the outdoors felt even better.

Moments like these were common. My classroom would have been Vicki's worst nightmare. She would have told me to avoid this much noise at all costs. Now I found myself surrounded by light and sound, two things that wore me out more than anything else.

No amount of training or number of textbooks on effective pedagogy could have prepared me for the real classroom either. I hit a learning curve like a bowl of jelly hits a roller coaster. I had to know how to best organize papers, when to give out homework, what homework to give, how to effectively separate the talkers, how to discipline the talkers, and how to keep my students from stealing my school supplies. I was overwhelmed by the surrealism of it all.

Yet I loved my student teaching semester more than I loved most things. It reminded me that I had a purpose in life. And most importantly, that I could pursue it despite my brain injury. I worked harder than I ever knew I could. And for free. I was paying for it, actually. About two thousand dollars. I told my students this once as I was handing out birthday donuts that I couldn't afford.

"Sorry, dears," I said. "You get half a donut. Maybe someday when I am getting paid to teach, you can find me and I'll give you a full one." I chuckled as I halved two boxes of chocolate glazed.

"What do you mean, Ms. H?" Bella shouted.

"You don't get *paid* to teach us?" Jonathan chimed in.

Lindsay smiled and gently explained that I was paying the university to be a teacher for a semester. Their jaws dropped to the floor alongside their half donuts. It made no sense to them that someone would put themselves through such a thing: paying for hours upon hours of labor with no monetary reward.

The reward I experienced was certainly my students and the chance to watch them grow. I couldn't have gone into teaching if I didn't love my kids. They were bright and funny, dedicated, and sometimes sleepy. I reveled in my new identity as Mother Hen. If one of my students was bullied in class, I was ready to take the punch or the insult. If somebody was failing math with Mr. So-and-So, I was learning pre-calc. It was the most challenging and worthwhile experience of my life.

Those six months of student teaching were a whirlwind. I wanted to write all of it down, but I barely had creative juices to spare by the end of the school day. When I did find time to write on the weekends, I felt guilty, like I should have been grading papers or planning. I considered starting a blog, but my portfolio deadline for the university was looming. Some days I was frantic. I caught myself in a daily battle of whether to write or whether to research whatever the hell I was supposed to be teaching the next day. Writing was the only thing that made sense anymore amid the confusion of being a teacher, and I didn't even have time to consider it. But when I could write, it provided me a sense of stability. I could control the words on the page, unlike the rowdy students in my classroom.

Even so, I ended up with this: a mere page of bullet points that can't be considered fully fleshed-out ideas. As I read them now, I'm not quite sure what they all mean, so I doubt you will either. Nevertheless, it was an important part of my life and recovery that shan't be forgotten. No, it *shan't*.

Here's the entirety of what I wrote during my student teaching semester in the spring of 2015:

- Brain stimuli: what science has to say about having too many tabs on your computer open.
- This job is like being on drugs. But they aren't fun, and I constantly feel like I'm tripping balls.
- So a kid made me cry today.
- March Madness: interview-mania.
- It's nice when it's raining, because then the sky is crying instead of me.
- Making coffee: the dos and don'ts.

- Cerebral cortex is still my safe word.

- I need a minute to process what the fuck is going on in my life.

- Shut your phone off for an hour, then watch it blow up with junk mail and creepy Tinder messages for a lifetime.

- "Wife Me" tattoo on forehead, and other frustrations with being an intense human.

- Daddy weight. Except I don't have a kid. And I'm also not a man.

- "Hey, you should hire me! I did great teaching a bunch of brain-damaged sixteen-year-olds in rehab!"

- My therapists probably think I'm dead by now.

- What would I do with a million dollars? Probably pay off my student loans and hire someone to massage my scalp every day.

- What the hell am I doing? And other questions I ask myself on a daily basis.

- How to disappoint your parents: tattoos and other questionable life decisions.

- No, really, Lindsay. Let me clean this coffee pot every day. It's the only thing in my life that I can control right now.

- The end of an era: being a clean person and why I can't seem to keep my clothes off the floor.

- What is income? And other things I don't know.

- Just ran into my brain surgeon in a pizza parlor. Damn, he is fine.

- What if I just sold this leftover Percocet to my friends? I'd make a killing.

- Nah, I like this Percocet. The Percocet can stay.

- What are the chances that this guy will take me on a second date if I tell him I used to be in a wheelchair?

- Why don't kids write their names on their papers? I mean, *for fuck's sake.*

- Someone from HealthONE just sent a photographer to take pictures of me teaching for a "Spalding success story." That sounds cool.

- That photographer from HealthONE just photoshopped a picture of my head onto a different picture of my body. That's not cool.

- The last day of school is June 6? Ah, hell no. I ain't about that life.

- There are absolutely no days off in April. But at least I can drink alcohol again.

As you can see, it was a dark time.

I learned more in six months of student teaching than I ever had in college or in quasi-adulthood. I grew immensely as a person. All my negative self-talk about my teaching future melted away. I was doing things I shouldn't have been able to do. Things I *hadn't* been able to do a few months before. And over time I finally cracked the code to teaching: care about your kids. That's it.

While content surely has its home in our history-loving hearts, kids aren't going to remember the intensity of the Civil War ten years from now. Shit, probably not even ten minutes from now. What they remember is your passion, your never-ending kindness. How excited you get when they walk in the door each day. They remember when you ask them how their grandmother is doing in the hospital. That you stayed after school for two hours so that they could take a makeup test. That's it. Just care about them. *Every. Single. Day.*

So I cared about them. And in return, I let those goofy, hormonal teenagers fill me with love, affection, and sometimes annoyance. They filled me up so much that I almost forgot about the hole in my head.

# Hi, I Have a Learning Duh-bility

Student teaching wasn't just about teaching my students. It was also about teaching myself. I learned how to make the perfect cup of coffee, how to spill that coffee down the front of my white blouse during fifth period, how to stay awake in an afterschool meeting, and how to regroup after falling asleep in an office chair during a fire drill. There was so much to learn about this place and so much to discover about me—and all the little ways my body tried to handle public school. Sometimes I couldn't handle it. Finally I broke.

Two months in, I curled up on my bed, writhing in emotional pain; I'd just snapped at my entire family at the dinner table. I'd been working myself into an anxious fury with my teaching portfolio, a requirement of my student teaching program and a monstrosity that involved deep analysis of my teaching practice, video of me teaching, and a miniature novel commenting on every choice I'd made in the classroom. It was the bane of my existence. A festering sore that left permanent scars on my psyche. To be fair, my portfolio does not deserve that poetic introduction. My portfolio was a pubescent asshole.

When I resumed my student teaching semester in January, I took a few weeks to get to know the kids again before I launched into a thorough portfolio panic. Being a full-time teacher was hard enough for my brain to navigate. But lesson planning and meetings and grading until late hours of the night began to stack onto my already weighed-down and gooey brain matter. I was unstable and emotional and fantastic. I was delightfully struggling and trying not to show it.

I flashed back to rehab often. I'd shown my therapists what I was expected to do for the portfolio to pass my student teaching semester. They laughed at me. They thought I was pulling their legs.

"Oh, Mimi!" Kendra said. "Someone recovering from a brain injury couldn't possibly get this done within that time frame. Good one though, Mimi. *Good one!*" I'd already been in panic mode before my injury. Now I was frantic on all cylinders.

I didn't hate the portfolio because it was a necessary step to getting my teaching license. I'm not talking about a logical assessment of my abilities as a future educator. This portfolio made no attempts at logic or reason. Its three lengthy tasks quite possibly contained more text than this lovely book. The written prompts required commentary on educational choices, which, by the way, is not a bad thing; educators, especially inexperienced ones, should analyze their own teaching practices. The problem was that the labor needed to complete the portfolio was so intensive that it would send teachers spiraling into hysteria, depression, and resentment, from which none of us fully recovered.

I wasn't just *teaching* for six months. I was grading papers and thinking and improvising and standing on my head and working my ass off and trying to impress everyone. I was waiting in line at the copy machine and going to meetings and making coffee runs and trying to get kids to like me or even respect me. I'd go to bed at five o'clock every night after a single glass of wine while covered in late work that I fell asleep trying to enter into the electronic grade book.

I could feel my brain matter tightening uncomfortably. I was sure this was the quickest way to end up back in Dr. Crawford's office. Which maybe wouldn't have been so bad, since he was such an attractive man. But my brain couldn't prioritize information. Just months earlier I'd had to choose between stimuli like lights and sounds. Talking to someone with music on in the background was a no-go. Writing down a phone number with the lights on simply didn't happen. Our brains are wired to zero in on what's important—when they're functioning, that is. Now I was tasked with prioritizing complex layers of stimuli and information and expected to function like an adult, all the while juggling the side effects of my brain injury.

It's amazing how many things going on at once we learn to ignore in order to cope in society. I'm typing this sentence sitting in a coffee shop. It's raining outside. I'm surrounded by fizzing espresso machines, lively conversations, and the low hum of my computer. Light music is playing from the stereo to my left. Someone behind me keeps sniffling. I just burned my tongue on my tea. I can't believe how hard my brain is working to master the task of writing a complex paragraph amid this chaos. It's probably not that great a paragraph, but still. The brain is a marvelous machine, an intricate and all-knowing organ. But during times of stress, like recovering from a cavernous angioma, the brain needs a little help.

My face swollen and my nose plugged up with snot, I dialed Riley's phone.

"It's like every day is a marathon," I sobbed. "I don't know if I can get through this okay." I felt like a rug had been pulled out from beneath me. All that was being asked of me was suddenly too much. I cursed my damaged brain and its inability to focus on anything for longer than two minutes. By the end of an average teaching day, I'd lost the ability to communicate my feelings or thoughts to those around me, and I wasn't even teaching a full load of classes. The deadline for my portfolio was daunting; my fate seemed dismal. I'd been tasked with the impossible, expected to organize a massive amount of material and convert it into something meaningful. Some days I thought it would be easier to quit and go to clown school. Some days I wondered if I would survive.

"I guess this is what it feels like to live with a learning duh-bility..."

I stopped for a second to contemplate what had come out of my mouth—a deliriously funny joke that my brain had played on my unsuspecting awareness. "I meant *disability*! Learning disability!"

Riley and I burst into laughter, and we kept going for what felt like hours.

After my phone call with Riley, I came to terms with my limitations. I needed to focus if I was to make it through my student teaching alive. And for that I needed help.

My dad pulled out the gigantic whiteboard from the garage; this was a relic from my childhood days, back when we kids had complex extracurricular schedules. Each member of the family received a different color dry-erase marker. My dad would draw up a calendar, complete with neat boxes and a legend with our colors. This made it easy to tell, on any given night in a four-month period, what each of us would be doing and where. Killin' it, parents.

"Break it into manageable pieces," Dad said softly as we hauled the dusty whiteboard into the dining room. "Make a system that works for your brain."

We cleaned it off, and I began figuring out how my new brain operated in this uniquely frustrating environment. I wanted to make this whole life thing easier to process and prioritize. I needed to help my brain navigate all the overlapping shit I was trying to do at once.

I marked off a space on the whiteboard for a monthly calendar. I copied down all my important due dates for student teaching. I color-coded. Sticky notes that had previously been crammed in my teaching bag were transferred to the board. I added a to-do list down the side, with big black boxes that I could check off once I'd accomplished a task. And I made lists for everything. I had a list of which lists I was going to use, and each list contained an extensive list of directions for using it. I am *listless* just thinking about it all. Ha. I'm funny. Add that to the reasons you're reading this book. It's a lengthy list, I'm sure.

I finished a preliminary organizational system for the board and stepped back and sighed heavily. I was thankful that Dad had suggested this. I could breathe a little easier, breathe without feeling like the world was crashing in on me like a gnarly Willis car accident.

Luckily for me, I have techniques to overcome the struggles that accompany my brain injury. I can create a quiet and safe space; I can use planners and reminders. I can meditate. I am equipped to practice these techniques successfully most days. This is not the case for many.

Recovering reasoning and organization functions can feel impossible for someone recovering from a brain injury. Making grocery lists, going to the store to get the items, and following a recipe require a tremendous amount of focus from the brain. This was something I'd always taken for granted.

I will never forget the first moment I didn't feel like myself, when I was no longer the me I thought I knew. I was with my mom out for a day of shopping pre-surgery. By this point I was losing the ability to use the left side of my body and walked with a slow drag. My vision was almost entirely double; I got dizzy every time I moved my head.

Our first stop was the Kohl's department store to look for clothes. Mom was probably trying to get me out of the drool-stained sweatpants I had been wearing since the first hospital visit weeks prior. She's adorable. I love her.

I couldn't manage to put the clothes on in the changing room, so Mom had to help me. I'd never been helpless like that. We hobbled over to the register to purchase a blue blouse, and I pulled out my phone to send a Snapchat. Probably something to the effect of "Mall Excursions with Mom," with a video of me going spelunking through the aisles, running into clothing racks.

As I closed one eye to send the video without my double vision messing me up, I noticed the clerk watching me. I transitioned my shifty eyes to look back at him. Eye contact was hard. It took me a few seconds, and I got dizzy, but I managed to look the man in the eye.

"You doin' okay there?" he asked.

"Yeah, sorry," I said. "It's just my brain injury." I focused my attention back on my phone.

"Oh yeah? Is your brain injury from using your phone too much?"

"Nope. Just your run-of-the-mill cerebral hemorrhage!" I said with a big jerk smile.

My mom added politely that it was "our field trip out," and I slunk out of the store, feeling ridiculous. Of course the man hadn't meant to bring the reality of my disability into full light. And of course my brain swelling had impacted the rational part of my brain, the part in control of appropriate social behavior. But I still felt stupid.

We continued our journey to Panera Bread. While I wasn't excited about having one more person point out how brain-dead I looked, I could at least get a bread bowl.

The place was packed. It was the loudest room I had ever experienced. People barked orders and moved tables, machines beeped, and music played over top of it all. Was this a Panera Bread or a NASA launchpad? "Can we just go?" I kept my wonky eyes on the floor and avoided haphazard eye contact with anyone.

We ordered our food as quickly as we could, and I focused on how soon I could obtain my mac and cheese bread bowl and get the *hell* out of there before somebody who knew me spotted my skinny legs dragging on the floor.

When we got home, I felt as though I had just run a marathon. Now I understand why the simple task of shopping for a blouse and a bread bowl became so overwhelming. My executive functioning was shot to hell. I couldn't prioritize stimuli, so every sound and movement set me off. This can be a lifelong struggle for someone with a brain injury. And most of the time we look perfectly functional on the outside.

While the lasting effects of my injury are minimal and manageable, I recognize that not all people are so lucky. The hemorrhage could have left me blind, permanently disabled, or dead. I cry at least three times a week thinking about this. When I drive my car. As I type on my computer right now. When I look outside and realize that I can differentiate shapes and colors and make sense of them too. Good *god*, I could be blind right now. Had things been a millimeter or so to the left or right, I would most certainly not be sitting here in my classroom, simultaneously monitoring my students and secretly writing my book.

I am blessed, and I am humbled. When things don't go my way or I am frustrated by some menial life happenstance, I must remember this: Today I am living with a learning duh-bility. And today I am alive.

## Scar Tissue

Every so often I run my hand across my scar and scratch it. It itches frequently, so this happens a lot, actually. When I do this, I not only set in motion a long fit of scratching but also reminisce about what I went through to get that scar. Sometimes I find myself in denial that I ever had to relearn how to walk. I seem to forget the hospital beds and anxiety. Then I feel the goofy hair growing back, scratch my scalp, and take a deep breath. I am forced to confront my scar every day—and the pain and the love that accompany it.

This is a good thing. Fear of pain is worse than the pain itself. That's why our bodies, and with effort our hearts, forget pain, or try. They forget pain so that we can survive, because if we never forgot, we'd never leave our homes, and we'd certainly never birth children. The human race simply couldn't sustain itself. And after a while it gets easier to live with these blemishes. Scars become more like friendly souvenirs that say, "Please don't do that again" or "You're a goddamn idiot for trying to jump over that fence in a miniskirt." They don't wreck your life so much anymore if you put in the time to tend to them, which can be painful too.

Because not all scars are visible. Some scars exist only in the fabric of our being, hidden from the naked eye. Sometimes we get hurt, and it leaves a mark.

I got my first heart scar with James. It still itches just like my head, and occasionally I must come face to face with my heart's painful journey too. It can happen easily enough; an old camera in an antique store, a flannel shirt, a forgotten painting, each can bring out a different and forgotten emotion. But whether it's joy or remorse, I sigh and realize I have a long way to go. Maybe I don't want to fully let go; perhaps I run my hand across my scars because it's too painful to walk away completely.

It's not like this shit's easy. Acknowledging scars is the first step in what's likely a 237 million-step stairway to healing. I was hesitant about even making that first step. I tried running around my problems with all kinds of quick fixes and fake solutions. I was convinced I knew how to go about curing myself.

Less than a month after the breakup, I met some of my friends for a girls' night downtown. We sat in my friend Maisie's living room and devoured a jumbo box of wine as I tried to make sense of what was going on. I wanted to get past my heartache, but I didn't know the first thing about my heart. So I'd brought a secret weapon—something I hoped would empower me.

"You brought a box made of Lego?" Lexi placed her glass of wine on the counter. "Is this your coping mechanism? I mean, I guess everyone's got their thing."

It was a Lego radio. James had made it for me during our first year together; that was the year of handmade gifts. He had taken out the parts of a working radio and put them inside Lego. It was fully functional and had been sitting in my room since the breakup, taunting me.

"Let's destroy the *shit* out of this thing," I slurred while juggling the radio with my wine glass.

"Alley way," Maisie said. "Let's do this."

The girls chanted, "Do it, do it, break that box. Do it, do it, *break that box!*" as we lugged it downstairs and out into the street. Temptation pulsed through me like the sugar rush from XL Pixy Stix. I also felt ceremonious, so I took a minute to collect my thoughts as Lexi shouted, "Speech!"

I hadn't prepared a speech. But I knew exactly what I wanted to say.

"This is for that time," I said, swinging the radio by the cord. "When we're both forty-five, and I run into you on the street." I was building energy now and swinging the radio madly, my voice growing. "And I've got a cute kid and a hot-ass husband, and I am *successful as fuck*." I was screaming, powerful like a Mommy Gorilla. "And you are bald and fat and alone and still living at home with your mother!"

I slammed the Lego radio down with the might of a thousand Chuck Norrises, and the crowd went wild.

I was magnificent and power-hungry. I stomped on the pieces and danced around them in my drunken bliss as the girls joined in. I wanted desperately for James to see me curb-stomping his radio. This was what healing was, I thought. *This is how you heal your heart.* I wanted him to feel my heels digging into every—

My power trip ended in fifteen glorious seconds. A woman barged out of her home across the street. "I will call the cops immediately if you don't pick up every piece of that Lego radio!"

Okay, so she didn't know it was a Lego radio. She thought it was glass. Because it makes more sense that a bunch of adults would be smashing lightbulbs in the street instead of a giant block of Lego. Had she known the importance of me smashing the daylights out of that thing, she might have been kinder to us. But not likely. Apparently people had small children in the neighborhood, including her.

As we shamefully picked up thousands of small Lego pieces, we tried to explain that I was really the victim here, but we were really sorry about making the mess, and there was no need to call the authorities, really, because we were sorry, *oh god are we sorry*.

We finished cleaning up our mess, and I half laughed, half cried my way to the sofa. That rush of power had been so quickly put out by adult responsibility and the phrase "this is not a frat house." She said that. I laughed, thinking about whether people went to frat houses to smash Lego around and make gallant monologues. I thought that was the kind of frat house I would like to join someday.

I could laugh all I wanted, but I'd taken one step forward and two steps back. I thought I was on the road to recovery. Really, I was just getting started. I didn't understand healing at all. And as long as I kept doing it my way—catapulting myself recklessly into new relationships—my scar would continue to rip open at the seams.

# Get Thee to a Nunnery

I was raised Catholic. I know about communion. I know how to eat the body of Christ without making a mess of myself. And I know about nuns. The first thing I learned as a kid was their knack for torturing my father in primary school and turning rulers and pencils into weapons of mass destruction. I also knew about *Sister Act* and the infamous nun habit that made Whoopi Goldberg perpetually cool in my eyes.

When I chose the College of Saint Benedict for my first year of college, I found out a bit more. And though the nuns did not resemble Whoopi in their nun gear, they were awesome. They welcomed the first years in the Great Hall, like at Hogwarts. They blessed our journeys. Some of them were even professors.

*Man, Sister Margaret Catherine is really bustin' my balls with this research paper right now...*

When I returned home to Colorado, I left my nuns in the monastery. Years went by, and I hardly remembered a time once existed when I lived among nuns.

Then I saw her.

I saw her while jogging in my parents' neighborhood one afternoon in the summer after my student teaching. My brain was still healing, but I was well on my way and preparing for my first real job post-injury. The nun was decked out to the nines—habit, prayer beads, veil, all of it. *A nun in the hood.* And I had spotted her in plain sight, a refreshing memory of days past.

I can't put my finger on why I adore nuns so much, but I do. They put me at peace. They are quiet and all-knowing. They speak the truth, and they've got great style. And it's not just the habit that draws me to mysterious and elusive neighborhood nuns. It's the no-*nun*-sense principles. See what I did there? I made a *nun*. Like a pun…with a nun. Nun pun. Anyway.

The summer after student teaching was a troubling time for me emotionally. I could feel myself slipping into muggy confusion, attempting to find love the wrong way yet again. In May I hit my one-year anniversary of being dumped, and I left the classroom the following month, dazed and confused. I had no idea what I was doing with my life. Test-driving adulthood seemed as scary as my first post-brain drive with Mom to the pottery class. I was alone and covered in emotional scar tissue. So I got back into online dating.

For a few months I went on more random dates, always coming home disappointed. The men I dated were either awkward with strange personalities or devastatingly handsome and interesting. I gave them names like Pizza and a Sunburn, Evil Twin, and Coffee Snob. Sometimes they'd fall for me, and I'd want nothing to do with them—or vice versa. We'd never be on the same page. I felt like Dorothy on her never-ending quest to get back home, constantly encountering strange groupies and being unable to shake them. But at least Dorothy had cool shoes.

On July 5, 2015, I went on a date with a young man named Henry. Devastatingly handsome and interesting, he was tall, Argentinian, and in a band, and had tattoos. He was by far the most striking man I had ever been on a date with. A real date. Not just me throwing a napkin at his face or sending him postcards from a thousand miles away. As conversation flowed easily, we ordered beer after beer and discussed our travels, current political scandals, and my recent medical history.

That bit told me I liked him. While I freely broadcasted my brain injury to the world, I would only tell a guy about my brain on a first date if I truly liked him. Like really *liked him* liked him.

We laughed together and walked the few blocks to his apartment. He played me a song that he'd just written for guitar. I swooned into his leather furniture. When he finished his song, he sat next to me on the couch, inching closer and closer, but it wasn't creepy like it had been with Creepy Face-Holding Guy, because I was super into it. And if he'd wanted to make me into a lampshade, then for sure he'd have done it already.

There we were, happily shootin' the what-have-you and making out like champions, and an awful thought crossed my brain waves: *He's never going to talk to you again.* I pushed the thought back to the messed-up part of my brain. You know, the part that was just operated on a second ago.

It was getting late, so I asked Henry to walk me back to my car. He obliged. But I was terrified. Even after hours of laughter and some primetime great kisses from Henry the Argentinian, I was in torment. *He's never going to talk to you again.*

A day went by, and he hadn't texted me back yet. Because he was camping with his dad. He had told me about this before I left his apartment that night. But it didn't matter. *I am garbage. I am garbage. I am garbage.* I repeated this phrase over and over for the next twenty-four hours. I wasn't even good enough for myself; how could I be good enough for Henry the fucking handsome Argentinian?

After a few days of agony, I set fire to my own happiness. I took a match and some lighter fluid to any chance I had at romance with Henry.

The past year of my life caught up with me in a very big way. The extensive line of make-believe relationships and fake Prince Charmings came flooding back like a familiar brain bleed. James had left me for someone else. Secret Agent Man had ghosted after a wedding invitation. The Canadian had a Canadian girlfriend. The list seemed endless. I felt so small and paper thin. *I am garbage*—it finally made sense. It wasn't just a phrase in a fortune cookie. I took it as the absolute, irrefutable truth.

I sent Henry a defensive text message outlining my discontent with the male species, thinking that I had saved myself from future heartbreak. I thought I was being smart by protecting my heart and my head. I thought I was being Beyoncé.

Several hours later he responded in disbelief. He told me his phone had died while he was camping and that he'd just gotten home. He was shocked at my behavior and hurt that I had jumped to such conclusions. He said we would not be hanging out again. When I read the text, my heart fell out my butt and onto the carpet. I was crushed. I sent myriad apologies and tried to explain that I'd been burned so many times that I didn't realize what I was saying.

Finally, after taking a serious and painful look in the mirror, I reached out to some friends to talk sense into me. One of my favorite friends and old roommates, Gina, had seen me at my worst after James. She'd force-fed me toast and jam. She'd tried to give me advice then too, though I'd been unable to take it in at the time. But I thought she'd know what to say now, and she did.

She freaking killed it.

"Mercy, grace, and forgiveness," she said, looking intently into my eyes and away from the cupcake that surely must have been more important than my dating woes.

"*Mercy* is when you don't give someone what you know they deserve," she said. "If you broke my one-million-dollar vase, I could give you mercy by telling you that I'm going to replace it and not make you pay for it.

"*Grace* would be if I tell you that it's okay that you broke the vase and that I still love you. And *forgiveness* is when I take the pain that I know I should put on you and I put it on myself. Maybe I should be upset that you broke my vase, but instead I'm going to take the pain for me and decide to forgive you."

*Decide. She said decide.* A million times I heard the word ring loudly in my frontal lobe. *Wait. I get to decide things now?* The idea that I could just decide to change my fairy-tale brain and join my new reality seemed so simple, so obtainable. Crap on a cracker, why hadn't I thought about this before?

"You're not crazy, Mimi." She squeezed my hand tight. "When we get hurt, we hurt others," she said, all Gene Wilder when he's super-wise and shit in that chocolate factory because he knows things. "It's natural, actually. Forgiveness is the weird thing. Forgiveness is not natural."

It was all starting to click in my mooshy mind.

"You can decide to forgive him, and all of them. It will hurt, because you must take that pain and put it on yourself. But you can decide. You can decide to forgive *yourself.*"

Mercy, grace, forgiveness. I had to give myself these things. And this is where the nuns come back in.

As Gina and I parted in the misty streets of Denver that night, I announced to the neighborhood, "Get thee to a nunnery!" I screeched it into the stars.

I said this because Hamlet said it to Ophelia. And while Hamlet was kind of a whack job, his suggestion that Ophelia put herself away for a while rang true. I needed to take a step back. Not just from dating and relationships, but from myself. I wanted to find myself again, to start over. I wanted to love myself free of another person. I wanted to embrace my scars, every one, just for me.

After Henry the Argentinian, I decided to put myself away for a while. I got myself to a nunnery. I mean, not literally. I'd have to go back to the Midwest for that sort of thing, and I really don't enjoy the wind chill.

But I took a step back. I assessed the true and beautiful dysfunction of my life. I wasn't sure if I would ever find love again. I wasn't even sure anymore that I knew what love was.

I used to force the kind of love I thought I wanted. I'd stack up my expectations nice and high for James so that he was sure to fall short, no matter what. The heating pad incident was only one example, and it wasn't about the heating pad at all; it represented something I desperately needed that James was unable to give me at the time. But life has shown me that I can find this kind of love in many forms. I have seen it in my father when he spends hours cooking my favorite meals without being asked. I have seen it in my mother when she shows up to my comedy shows even when she's exhausted from a twelve-hour work day. I have seen it in my brother when he microwaved a bag of rice for me every single day for months, and in my sister when she gives me hugs even though she dislikes touching people. I have seen it from countless friends and family who have put my happiness above their own in my time of need.

And most of all I have seen it in myself. After all was broken and frail, I have seen the love that I can give to my own head and heart.

For me to be truly happy, I need to change my fantasy brain into a nun brain. I need to simplify in there—it's too fucking complicated in that gooey thing. If nuns live in poverty, chastity, and obedience, then my brain must get rid of those fancy princess shoes and castles. My brain should be pure and unsullied by the temptation to stay clueless about intimacy and relationships. And for the love of all that is holy and nunlike, my brain needs to listen to my heart, to know when it's taking things too far. My brain also needs to be Sister Bertrille in *The Flying Nun*. Just fucking awesome, that's what.

The process of changing my brain won't be easy. I don't have the tools for this kind of thing. But if I want to be happy, then I will have to figure it out. I'm pretty sure this will be the most crucial decision of my life. That, and stalking the local nun in my neighborhood.

## Remission

I had a dream many years ago. In the dream I was ten years old. I was at a masquerade ball and was decked to the nines in a seventeenth-century ballgown and a wig. I sat on a bench looking out onto the dance floor, probably searching for some prepubescent boy to dance with. I considered leaving the dance floor and relocating to the cheese tray. But right as I was about to make a move for the Gouda, a woman approached me.

She was in her mid-thirties, with a blinding white wig. She wore a mask covered in jewels and lace, but through the holes in the mask I could see that her eyes were a magnificent blue, sparkling under the light of the chandelier. Her dress was more complex than mine. It was a royal red and billowed down to the floor, and it had black trimmings. She wore a corset too and even had the boobs to fill it out. I shifted, uncomfortable. All the places that this random woman could sit, and she plunks herself down next to me? Freaking weirdo. I eyed the cheese tray but sat still, waiting for the woman to make a move or at least offer me some spiked punch from inside her corset.

For thirty seconds we sat in silence. Me and the boobed lady. Then she turned to me and took off her mask, and I gasped. It was me. A thirty-something, boobed version of me!

"It's okay, it's just me," Wise Me said.

I squirmed on the bench. The cheese tray was dead to me. I had learned how to time travel! And I had boobs! I opened my mouth to ask the million and one questions flying through my head, but no sound would come out. *Do we get married? Is he totally hot? What job do we have now? Is our Game Boy going to be worth anything in the future?* Wise Me raised her hand to silence me, even though I wasn't actually speaking.

"We're going to be okay," Wise Me said. "We're going to be just fine."

I sat for some time with the older and wiser version of myself. I was tempted to ask questions; I wanted to know the future. I wanted to know *my* future. But we just existed in silence. I still didn't know if I would ever have a hot husband or if I'd get to sing and dance on Broadway like I'd dreamed of as a kid, but Wise Me had promised I was going to be okay.

There are many ways to interpret dreams. No offense to Freud, but I don't think it means I'm into anything *that* obscene. I think about this dream a lot these days and wonder if it was a sign that I longed to be reassured even then. Throughout my life I have often questioned if I'm going to make it through; if I'm going to be okay. But I always am. No matter how stressed or horrible the situation, I've made it out okay in the end. And we all do, one way or another.

Remission is easy to slip into. We slide back to the anxiety, emotions, or dark memories that we wish we could forget. Friends and family are often astonished at my ability to fall into thought patterns that are not healthy for me. But it's okay to regress, and it's okay to have a few slip-ups here and there. Nobody is perfect. And life can balance us back without us even realizing it. We don't have the luxury (yet) of being able to ask our future selves to reassure us, but somehow things fall into place and save us at the last second.

I never did ask my future self if I'd have a brain hemorrhage. At age ten I probably didn't even know I had a brain. My questions centered on the healthy relationships that I saw among my parents and family. It's what I always have and always will want in life: to feel loved and reassured, to know someone loves me despite my flaws. When I saw my older self, I was astonished and proud. Not only was I a knockout with fully developed breasts, but I was wise and worldly.

Maybe the dream meant nothing. After all, my boobs are still relatively small, and I doubt they'll get any bigger at this point. But maybe it meant everything. Maybe my brain was trying to tell me something, leave miniature breadcrumbs for me to find throughout my life. I may not have seen these breadcrumbs while smashing the Lego radio in the alley. I may not have seen them on the cold examination table when the nurse told me that my brain was bleeding. But boy, do I see them now. And I'm gonna eat them up.

## The Monster at the End of This Book

*Thursday, September 17, 2015, 9:11 p.m.*

Writing this sentence took five minutes. Or is it 5 minutes? I'm not a writer, I'm a teacher. I don't have time to argue. Writing this sentence took five minutes because I was knee-deep in grading Civil War essays, and I kept misplacing my favorite teaching pen. It took five minutes because I was too busy trying to eat a sandwich while simultaneously filling out my rental application for the studio apartment I plan on moving into next week. It took a year to write this sentence, this paragraph, and this story.

My favorite story as a child was *The Monster at the End of This Book*. In it a lovable and worried *Sesame Street* character named Grover tries to convince you not to turn to the next page for fear of a terrible monster at the end of the book. The guy tries everything—ropes, bombs, brick walls—to keep you from turning that damn page. I remember that as a child I'd force my mother to pretend the pages were heavy, weighed down by the brick. She needed superhuman strength to overcome Grover's obstacles.

Grover is a really determined dude. He does *not* want you to turn that page. And you just won't listen. Every time you disappoint him by grasping the page between your fingers, he urges you again to beware. I'd been wondering what all the hype was about the page turning, so I dug through the basement to find the book and read it again. I sat down on my parents' familiar red couch with some leftover pizza. *C'mon, Grover. What's the big deal?*

As Grover quickly realizes, the name of the book is *The Monster at the End of This Book*, and he's really scared of monsters. Grover tries to explain this fear as if it will be enough for you to respect his wishes and just walk away. But you don't do that. You turn the page again, like a big jerk. Because you think Grover's fear of monsters is kind of hilarious.

Grover breaks out some ropes to tie the pages together, but Mom's superhuman strength broke through those easily when I was a kid, and I channel her now as I push past the ropes and onto the next page. Again Grover is dissatisfied with the results. So now he nails the pages together and says something like "Do *not* turn the page! There is a monster at the end of this book!"

Unfortunately the nails were no match for my mother's guns back in the day. I take out my imaginary hammer now and unstick the nails from the pages while balancing my pizza in my mouth.

By this point Grover is agitated and worn out from trying to stop me from getting through to that monster. Grover thinks maybe a brick wall is the answer, but this doesn't seem to be a problem for my determined and greasy fingers.

We're nearly to the end of the book now, and Grover's just begging me to stop all this tomfoolery. "Please do not turn the page," he says. "Please. Please. Please."

As I sit on the couch today reading this book, I think it's very nice that he said please. I consider my next move. He did ask politely. But Mom and I turned the page anyway back then, and I turn the page again now. Because it seems awfully silly not to read a book that someone—probably not me—paid for. I hold the page tightly between my fingers, moving it as slowly as if it really weighed a thousand pounds. I lift the page to the other side with a deep sigh. *Oof, that was hard.* I search for the monster that will inevitably eat me, but it turns out that the monster at the end of the book is just Grover: a friendly and hairy little blue guy who wouldn't hurt a mosquito. If any of us feared the ending, we shouldn't have. Grover is adorable.

I'm not afraid of monsters, even scary ones. But I am terrified of ending this book.

Because ending something is always more difficult than beginning it. The moment you first see the pastry you are about to devour is always better than the moment you realize you are taking your final bite. Licking the spoon is only fun when there's more batter in the bowl. It's just pastry science. Therefore I'm having a tough time saying goodbye.

And like our friendly and off-kilter *Sesame Street* Grover, I would do anything to keep you from finishing this book. The truth is, I've been on this journey for so long that it seems a little wrong to walk away now. Like Grover, I'm afraid of myself. I'm afraid of who I am, or who I am not. I'm scared that I will look in the mirror after all this and not like what I see. So I carry a giant bag of ropes and TNT around to keep myself from truly confronting that image on the other side. I wonder if I've changed enough to pull myself out of my web of delusions. I fear that I haven't cast aside my noodly rowboats—that I'm still knee-deep in a sea of imagination and fake truths.

Confronting my delusions has always been hard for me. It was hard for me when I got dumped, it was hard for me when my health went south, and it's hard even now. I allowed my neurons to wrap themselves up in little knots, and eventually one of those knots stuck together and filled up with some blood. Maybe it needed to happen this way for me to face my skewed sense of reality. It's difficult looking back now to tell if I've done the right thing. It's hard to know if my surgery really rewired my inability to love myself and to make my own path. Because even when all the stitches had healed, I was left with more healing to do on my own. And after all this roller-coaster-style learning and fixing, I'd like to know if I'm better now than I was at the start of it, when I buckled myself in for the bumpiest ride of my life.

I'd tie your hands together to keep you from turning this page. It's a terrifying thought that not only could I walk away unchanged from this journey, but you could walk away from this book the same person as you were before. We could both keep making the same mistakes in love and in life and tell ourselves that we never need stray from the comfortable and easy. That's why Grover is so scared. He's terrified of facing himself, of asking the hard questions: *Am I a monster? Did I do the right things in this life?*

But maybe I don't have to be so afraid of the end. After all, the monster at the end of Grover's book is adorable, and we can safely assume from his kind smile that he pays his taxes on time and recycles. Maybe I can simply finish this book and acknowledge the journey for what it was—be proud of myself and move forward. I can take some bricks down from the walls I've built around my heart and be vulnerable for a while. I can take a break from trying to be a perfect checklist person and just be my goofy blue Grover self. I will keep making mistakes and learning from them. I will grow into my new life after heartbreak and hemorrhaging.

It's important I understand that what I'm growing toward is awesome. Despite the stress-induced panic that accompanies me almost daily, having the opportunity to be alive in the first place is altogether badass. I survived the classroom several times, once with a brain bleed and then again while my brain was on the road to healing. I have my own desk now with pencil shavings all over it and am learning new things about my students and myself every day. I juggle my hectic work life while occasionally dipping my baby toe back into the dating pool. I don't picture Prince Charmings as much as before and am okay with just getting some free cheese dip and calling it a day if I don't feel like pursuing it. I run half marathons, and I get a new bruise every hour by bumping into desks in my classroom. When I look back on this day a year ago, I can hardly believe how far I've come. Well, literally not far at all. I'm still sitting on the same couch that I started this book on. Sorry, ruined the moment.

I wasn't always brave. I was like Grover once, scared of myself. I hid in corners during weddings, wishing that James would fall back in love with me. I feared letting myself feel the pain of my heart and head injuries, so instead I just made them the butt of a joke. I did it to make fun of myself, to point my finger at the mirror and emotionally harm my own existence. I wasn't always there for myself like I should have been, and for a while I really might have been a monster, forever leading myself down a path of unhappiness and self-doubt.

My friends and family tried to help me feel my pain for what it was. They wanted me to respect it—to take it seriously. I laughed at many of them for feeling my hidden hurt. I made fun of humans or animals who were scared, because it felt safer than admitting to myself that I was frightened of meeting my maker. I was afraid of dying alone, too young to have fully lived. But the fear didn't go away once I survived the initial trauma of brain surgery. Once I began to recover, I was afraid again, of not being myself anymore. I feared a change in the very basics of me, the way I walked, talked, and saw the world.

I never intended for any of this to happen. My year of brain bleeds and bad dates was not the romantic comedy that I'd cast myself in many times before. I'd pictured a life more Hollywood: James and I in our beautiful castle surrounded by water, with rowboats for our romantic evening outings. I'd imagined teaching being easy and that every child would become a better person for simply having met me. I pictured a lot of leisurely trips to the south of France, because teaching would pay me the big bucks. I certainly hadn't pictured my brain exploding while I ate cheese fries.

This book isn't perfect. And for once in my life, I can be okay with imperfect. I have to be now. With every well-planned part of my life, there is a mild to moderate hiccup: A casual tumble off a park bench while talking to my best friend, because I forgot to do my balancing exercises this week. A sentence that doesn't come out right because I've been teaching for four hours straight, and I don't think I've taken attendance yet, and at least twelve children in this room have asked me to use the restroom in the past thirty seconds, and did I just spill my coffee on my lesson plans *holy shit what is happening*. Executive functioning is hard and relationships are harder. My students love to point out my singleness daily.

"Miss, are you married?" a student will say.

"No sir. Now, how's that question on your paper coming?" I ask.

"But Miss, why?"

"Just a personal choice. Your answer to question two—"

"*Why are you all alone?*"

At this point in the conversation, I usually have to walk away before I end up in jail for smacking a kid with my yardstick.

But what my fourteen-year-old friend doesn't know is that I'm not alone. Not at all. It is because I am not alone that I have been able to tell this story. These are the things I hold on to, the people who carried me with gait belts and helped me successfully get my pants on again. The friends who set aside their busy lives to bring me cheeseburgers and the therapists who convinced me that I was brave. When some days felt impossible, they were there: my friends, my beloved family, and my smelly dog.

And I was there too; I chose to rewire my brain so that I could support my own self. So most of all I hold on to me. I hold on to my refusal to adhere to what people expect of me. I hold on to the sheer will that got me out of the wheelchair and into the hospital dining hall. And granted, Vicki may have yelled at me because I was supposed to take the wheelchair until I could walk—but damn it, I was determined to get to that salad buffet.

I owe my life to every human and earthly being who has smiled upon me with good grace during breakups, brain hemorrhages, and everything in between. And I owe it to myself. I know now that the only person who can repair the holes in my heart and my head is me; I am my own medicine.

I still make a lot of jokes today, funny ones, too. I tell jokes to crowds of strangers on weekends and to a room of thirty teenagers 7:30–3:30 Monday to Friday. I joke about my students and politics, and occasionally I'll tell a good period joke. Sometimes I make fun of myself, but with a new appreciation for what I've been through, for who I have been and for who I am now. I am both the scared and the confident Grover, reflecting on my life and journey as a new token of self-love and gratefulness.

There isn't a monster at the end of this book after all. It's just me—aged a few years and in a masquerade gown—telling you that I'm going to be okay. *drops mic*

The End

# Acknowledgments

When I first started writing this book, I had no idea how many thank you cards I'd have to write.

First and foremost, I would like to thank my beautiful and loving parents, John and Janet Gagnon. You weren't my first choice as I made my selection of human hosts from my spaceship, but I took a chance on you guys and it paid off. You are the most encouraging, selfless, humble people who exist. You saved my life and taught me all the right stuff. Sorry I put you through hell (and back) (like every day). I'm obsessed with the both of you.

In no specific order, I would like to thank some other people: Samantha Conway, for being the recipient of the terrible first draft and still my favorite roommate. Brennyn Buscarello, for being the first responder at every one of my life mishaps. You know all my urine-soaked secrets, and I'm so proud to call you my person.

I would like to thank Maurice Tucker for being there the whole time. Shout-out to Gina, Mel, Addie, and Maegan for holding me up during rough patches and force-feeding me. Alexis Pineiro, my Scurrbooboo, thank you for loving me at my lowest. You've never been above holding a pink wig out of my face as I vomited behind a dumpster, and I respect you for that.

Katrina McCarthy, for being there when I found out that I was scared and for seeing me through puberty. Your dedication to our friendship despite my horrible track record at answering your phone calls is truly revolutionary. Nancy and Kevin Massey, for trying to keep me as one of your own. My mother was a lot less worried when I was with you. The Ott family, you're so good to me. Karen Clancy, thank you for coming to my hospital room and giving me coffee when they wouldn't let me have it.

Big thanks to my Peanut, Melanie Rogers, who always believed in me. You are a beautiful gypsy soul, and your art will change the world. Ashlie Weisel, for being a ray of sunshine and for painting with me when I was losing motor function.

Jen Reiks, thanks for helping me learn how to use my hands again. The nursing and therapy staff of Saint Joseph Hospital and Spalding Rehabilitation Center, for putting up with my snarky remarks and showing me the greatest love I have ever known.

Rosie the chef extraordinaire, you are the hero of my story, and your smoothies are delicious AF.

I would like to thank East High School for your patience with me during student teaching. Jay Graham, for bringing me and all my friends plants that I sadly couldn't keep alive for very long. The Callahans, thank you for giving me a ton of snacks. Brittney Cortesy, for telling me my face wasn't fat (I know it was). I would also like to thank my "Brain Buddies" Joey Miyaki and Emily Wigstrom for letting me know I wasn't alone.

Shannon Connolly, without you I simply would not exist. This book wouldn't exist either. Because it was your idea. At least if I get sued, I can blame it on you. Attorney up, Croissant Rat! Jamie, thank you for telling me I was brave, even though I didn't believe you yet.

Kent Willmann, thank you for helping me be a damn good teacher. I would like to thank Jeanne Sparling for being the best. I would like to thank my nuggets Heather Claypool and Katie Currie for bringing me donuts in the ICU, which probably scared the shit out of you. I hope I didn't get any piss on your shoes. Kendra, thank you for your fun logic puzzles and games that helped me recover the messed-up parts of my brain.

I would like to give a special thank you to the entire cast of *'Til Death Do Us Party*:

you are the cutest murder mystery theater ever. Sorry for scaring the shit out of you on opening night. Emily Scraggs, thank you for being such a delightful human and friend to me and for letting my non-grandpa give you a pregnant flea plant. Lori, thank you for all that you did for me at Spalding Rehab; my recovery would not be possible without you. Dr. Todd Crawford, a gigantic shout-out to you for being such a spectacular neurosurgeon and for not shaving my entire head. I really appreciate that.

A special thank you to Erin Gagnon, for taking me on walks and for letting me be emotional. You are beautiful inside and out, and I'm so happy to call you my sister. Hayley Wagner, I would like to thank you for the purple hospital blanket and for being my friend back in Girl Scouts. I would like to thank Rebecca Garner for being such a stellar recovery buddy and bringing me Chipotle and cheeseburgers. Sylvia, thank you for helping me on the treadmill and for telling me to buy new shoes.

Brian, a.k.a. Bugger Boo, you are such a cool dude. You are so patient and kind, and my world is better because of you. Thank you, Miguel, for joking with me and making me feel like the most awesome patient at Spalding. I would like to thank Krista Gagnon for being a loving sister-in-law and helping pick out the elephant stuffed animal.

A huge shout-out to Vicki, my absolute favorite and a total pro at Wii Sports. Thank you for helping me walk over those stupid broomsticks, and sorry about that time I took my walker to breakfast instead of my wheelchair. Deana, you're cool too. Even though you stabbed me with needles. I would like to thank Audrey Sorensen for showing me the love that I needed and deserved.

I would like to thank everyone for the flowers that they gave me that I killed immediately. I would like to thank Auntie Doob, Auntie Di, Auntie Karen, Auntie Martee, and Auntie Janie for the chocolate, heating pads, and all the love. Lindsay, Tommy, and Parker Anderson, thank you so much for being amazing. And Linds, sorry about that one time I gave you a heart attack and almost died five days into the school year. I hope this does not discourage you from getting another student teacher. Thank you to Lois at Spalding Rehab, you made me me again.

Holy shit, and I would like to thank my dear friend Kristen Jorden for reading every stupid thing I have to say and pushing me to be a better teacher, writer, and human. You are everything I strive to be when I grow up, and I'm so happy that I met you, so that I can write your name here for you to see in print. *KristenJordenKristenJordenKristenJorden.*

I would like to thank my students, all three hundred or so of you from the past few years. You're all beautiful and annoying, and I want to adopt almost all of you.

Lastly, I would like to thank my editors and team: Carolyn Daughters and Brad Wetzler, for shaping this story. Christina Frey, you've taken my memoir game to a whole new level, and I am convinced you are my editorial soulmate. Howard Shapiro, thank you for taking a chance on me. Thank you all for your patience. Sorry it took me so long to finish this.

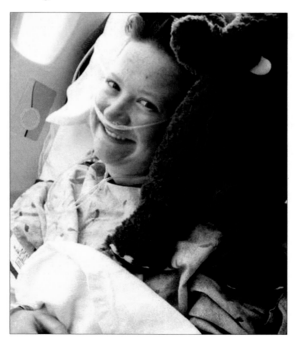

# About the Author

Mimi Hayes is an author, comedian, and curly-headed cartoon figure found on the back of napkins and old receipts. Originally from Denver, Colorado, she got her start in comedy by becoming a high school history teacher in a windowless classroom and getting heckled by teenagers. Mimi currently finds herself in New York City, writing, performing, and doing popsicle stick crafts with four-year-olds. She once built an IKEA bed all by herself and plans to open a puppy sanctuary in rural Connecticut when she's sixty-seven. You can cyberstalk her at mimihayes. com, follow her on Twitter (@mimihayesbrain1), or send her a carrier pigeon.